FIRST DO NO HARM

A PRACTICAL GUIDE TO MEDICATION
SAFETY AND JCAHO COMPLIANCE

Opus Communications
Marblehead, Massachusetts

First Do No Harm: A Practical Guide to Medication Safety and JCAHO Compliance is published by Opus Communications.

Copyright 1999 by Opus Communications, Inc.
Cover images ©1999 PhotoDisc, Inc.

ISBN 1-57839-035-4

Opus Communications provides information resources for the healthcare industry. A selected listing of our newsletters and other books is found in the back of this book. Arrangements can be made for quantity discounts.

Jennifer I. Cofer, Executive Publisher
Rob Stuart, Publisher
David Beardsley, Executive Editor
Kristen Woods, Executive Editor
Jean St. Pierre, Art Director
Mike Mirabello, Graphic Artist
Ian McLaughlin, Cover Designer
Deborah Cunha, Proofreader

Advice given is general. Readers should consult professional counsel for specific legal, ethical, or clinical questions. Opus Communications is not affiliated in any way with the Joint Commission on Accreditation of Healthcare Organizations.

For more information on this or other Opus Communications publications, contact:

Opus Communications
PO Box 1168
Marblehead, MA 01945
Telephone: 800/650-6787 or 781/639-1872
Fax: 800/639-8511 or 781/639-2982
E-mail: customer_service@opuscomm.com

Visit the Opus Communications World Wide Web site: www.opuscomm.com

Table of Contents

Acknowledgments

Opus Communications wishes to thank the following people for assisting in the development of this book:

Kenneth Barker, BS, MS, PhD
Department of Pharmacy
  Care Systems
Auburn University

David Bates, MD, MSc
Division of General Medicine and
  Primary Care
Brigham and Women's Hospital

Marcia Bowers, RN, MSN, CPHQ
Home Care Accreditation
  Consultant

Steven W. Bryant
Practice Director, Accreditation
  Services
The Greeley Company

Rick Croteau, MD
Executive Director for
  Strategic Initiatives
Joint Commission on Accreditation
  of Healthcare Organizations

Neil Davis, PharmD, FASHP
President
Safe Medication Practices
  Consulting, Inc.

**Elizabeth DiGiacomo-
  Geffers, RN, MPH, CNAA**
Healthcare Consultant

Sue Dill, RN, MSN, JD
Director of Health Policy
Ohio Hospital Association

Captain Charles R. Drew
Principal Research Scientist
NASA/ASRS Project

Michael Hirshland
Counsel to the United States
  Committee on the Judiciary
United States Senate

William Kelly, PharmD
Department of Pharmacy Practice
Mercer University

Lucian Leape, MD
Adjunct Professor of Health Policy
Harvard School of Public Health

Dennis Levin, MD, MPH
Director of Ambulatory Care
Harbor UCLA Medical Center

Katharine Luther
Director, Performance Improvement
Hermann Hospital

Ilene MacDonald
Executive Editor
Briefings on JCAHO

Rick McCumber
Director of Pharmacy
St. Joseph Regional Medical Center

Janet McIntyre
Media Relations Manager
Joint Commission on Accreditation
  of Healthcare Organizations

Carolyn Meier
Vice President for Learning Services
Management Prescriptives, Inc.

David Musa
Assistant Director of Pharmacy
University of Wisconsin Hospital
  and Clinics

Teresa Porrazzo, PharmD
President
Drug Therapy Consultants, P.C.

Donna Scott
Director of Quality Assurance
University Community Hospital

David Spencer
Chairman and CEO
Management Prescriptives, Inc.

Dennis Wallace, DABRM
Partner
Medical Risk Management
  Associates

Jack Zusman, MD
Professor, Florida Mental
  Health Institute
University of South Florida

Transforming Patient Safety

The credo "first do no harm" communicates one of healthcare's most powerful guiding principles: If medical treatment can't always make patients better, it certainly should not make them worse. But, at times, it does make them worse, and medication is often the reason why. One study suggests that as many as 1.3 million hospital patients each year are injured or killed during treatment, 19 percent of them (247,000 people) by medication.[1,2] Another study found that adverse drug reactions (ADR) could be the fourth leading cause of death in the United States.[3]

Beyond the human costs, there's the economic toll. A study by the Alliance for Aging Research places the annual cost of "medication misuse" at more than $100 billion; ambulatory care accounted for most of that total ($76.6 billion), while hospitals and nursing homes added $4 billion each.[4] The Harvard Medical Practice Study (see below, footnotes 1 and 2) reported similar findings with regard to hospital costs and estimated that patients foot a quarter of the bill ($1 billion). The

---

[1] *T.A. Brennan, L.L. Leape, N. Laird, et al, "Incidence of adverse events and negligence in hospitalized patients: results of the Harvard Medical Practice Study I," N Engl J Med 324: 370-6 (1991).*

[2] *L.L. Leape, T.A. Brennan, N. Laird, et al, "The nature of adverse events in hospitalized patients: results of the Harvard Medical Practice Study II," N Engl J Med 324: 377-84 (1991).*

[3] *Jason Lazarou, Bruce H. Pomeranz, and Paul N. Corey, "Incidence of Adverse Drug Reactions in Hospitalized Patients," JAMA 279 (15): 1204 (1998).*

[4] *Reported in: "Medication misuse in LTC costs $4 billion each year," McKnight's Long-term Care News, August 1998, 12.*

problem is so significant that a frank assertion by researcher David Classen almost seems too tame: "Drug use represents the most common intervention in medicine and has the potential for costly and deadly consequences."[5]

The healthcare industry has not ignored the potential risks of drug treatment. Key aspects of the licensing, training, and education requirements for caregivers—and of the laws, regulations, and accreditation standards that govern provider organizations—are meant to minimize those risks. But these intended safeguards exist within a culture that ultimately works against them. Healthcare and society tend to blame individuals for adverse events and outcomes, but a growing body of research suggests that systems are usually the problem, not people. Knowledge and intentions are important, but well-trained, well-intentioned individuals will sometimes fail when forced to contend with poorly conceived policies and procedures, defective or complex equipment, or an ineffective work environment. "The medical imperative is clear," a recent commentary argued; "to make health care safer we need to redesign our systems to make errors difficult to commit and create a culture in which the existence of risk is acknowledged and injury prevention is recognized as everyone's responsibility. A new understanding of accountability that moves beyond blaming individuals when they make mistakes must be established if progress is to be made."[6]

---

[5] David C. Classen, "Clinical Decision Support Systems to Improve Clinical Practice and Quality of Care," JAMA (editorial) 280 (15): 1360-61 (1998).

[6] Lucian L. Leape, David D. Woods, Martin J. Hatlie, Kenneth W. Kizer, Steven A. Schroeder, and George D. Lundberg, "Promoting Patient Safety by Preventing Medical Error," JAMA (editorial) 280 (16): 1444 (1998).

Redesigning the systems that govern medication use and conceiving a "new understanding of accountability" are tall orders. The latter, in particular, involves overcoming attitudes and modes of behavior that have become entrenched—almost instinctive—after decades of reinforcement. Healthcare professionals are told again and again that imperfection is inexcusable. Mistakes and preventable adverse events are treated as aberrations that call for aggressive training, punishment, or both. Organizations rarely address contributing systemic factors, which often lie outside the control of the "guilty" individuals. Attorneys, regulators, lawmakers, and society as a whole contribute to this atmosphere, demanding infallibility from healthcare professionals and often targeting them, not the systems in which they function, with legal or punitive action when they prove fallible. To err is human, we say, unless you work in healthcare.

But there are signs that the tide is turning. The people who want to change the way we think about safety and accountability in healthcare are finding an audience; more importantly, their proposals and hypotheses are being tested. This book examines those arguments as they apply to medication use, and it discusses relevant programs and initiatives:

- **Chapter 1, "A New Approach to Error Prevention,"** summarizes the arguments for redesigning systems and our understanding of accountability. It talks about relevant developments in other high-risk industries, like aviation, and it explores how those models might apply to healthcare and medication use.

- **Chapter 2, "Applying the Systems Approach: Models for Error Prevention,"** describes how the theories and views examined in

Chapter 1 are affecting medication use. It profiles organizations that are experimenting with new technologies and processes in an effort to improve the safety of drug treatment.

- **Chapter 3, "Performing a Root-Cause Analysis,"** explains healthcare's newest technique for responding to adverse events. Root-cause analysis is now required by the Joint Commission on Accreditation of Healthcare Organizations (JCAHO), in part because it shifts the focus of investigations from individuals to systems.

- **Chapter 4, "Designing and Implementing Improvement Proposals,"** addresses quality-improvement tools and techniques that will help organizations deal with the root causes and launch safety initiatives. Along with performance of root-cause analysis, this is a key requirement of the JCAHO's sentinel event policy and standards.

- **Chapter 5, "Complying with Relevant JCAHO Standards,"** gives an overview of JCAHO accreditation standards that apply to medication use and offers compliance tips. It also explores how the JCAHO standards are keeping pace with new strategies for preventing and responding to errors and adverse events.

Critics and skeptics may worry that this new approach to safety eliminates the notion of individual responsibility, but that argument misses the point. If individuals ignore policies, procedures, laws, and regulations—or if they lack necessary skills and knowledge—healthcare and society still have the means to respond. But it's easy to point fingers.

For years, healthcare organizations have failed to look beyond individuals to the systems that affect their ability to provide quality care. Indications that they may now be doing so signal a potentially important transformation. After years of telling people, "first do no harm," healthcare may finally be taking that safety directive to heart.

A New Approach to Error Prevention

Putting the issues in perspective

Imagine what would happen to the airline industry if nine or ten jumbo jets crashed each week, killing everyone aboard. People would probably stop flying. There would be hearings and lawsuits. The industry might be grounded. It might not survive. Yet, as Harvard researcher Lucian Leape, MD, has noted, that's what it would take for the number of annual plane-crash deaths in the United States to equal the estimated number of deaths caused by adverse reactions to medical treatment.[1]

Adverse drug events (ADE)—a blanket term that refers to preventable incidents (medication errors, drug interactions, etc.) and drug-induced complications that cannot be anticipated or prevented (e.g., unknown allergies)—are a leading cause of treatment-related death and injury. As many as 70 percent of them may be preventable.[2] Nonetheless, it appears either that ADE are becoming more common or that better reporting is revealing the true extent of the problem. One recent study, for instance, found that the number of annual deaths due to medication errors in the United States increased more than 250 percent between 1983 and 1993—from 2,876 to 7,391.[3] Another study found

---

[1] Lucian L. Leape, "Error in Medicine," JAMA, 272 (23): 1851 (1994).

[2] David W. Bates, David J. Cullen, et al., "Incidence of Adverse Drug Events and Potential Adverse Drug Events: Implications for Prevention," JAMA 274 (1): 29 (1995).

[3] David P. Phillips, Nicholas Christenfeld, and Laura M. Glynn, "Increase in U.S. medication-error rates between 1983 and 1993," Lancet, 351: 643-4 (1998).

that adverse drug reactions (ADR) may kill more than 100,000 people each year in the United States and could be anywhere from the fourth to sixth leading cause of death nationwide.[4] ADR, a narrower term than ADE, does not include errors made during drug treatment (e.g., wrong dose, wrong drug, missed dose, etc.).

The situation could, however, be worse; most medication errors do not harm patients. For instance, in a 1995 study, Dr. Leape and David Bates, MD, of Brigham and Women's Hospital in Boston, found that serious medication errors occurred in only about five out of every ten thousand doses administered to patients in two Boston hospitals.[5] So, it's important to remember that for each person who is harmed by medication, many more are helped.

Nonetheless, healthcare cannot afford to dismiss the problem of medication errors because most are relatively innocuous. Leape and Bates observed preventable ADE of varying severity, or potential ADE, in 7.3 percent of the patients involved in their study.[6] Other studies have estimated the medication-error rate at anywhere from 1.5 percent to 35 percent.[7] And when Bates and Leape extrapolated their data to determine hospital-wide totals, they estimated that 1900 ADE occur per year in each of the hospitals they studied.[8] That so few of the errors identified by Leape and Bates were serious is fortunate, but the relative

---

[4] Jason Lazarou, Bruce H. Pomeranz, and Paul N. Corey, "Incidence of Adverse Drug Reactions in Hospitalized Patients," JAMA 279 (15): 1204 (1998).

[5] Lucian L. Leape, David W. Bates, et al., "Systems Analysis of Adverse Drug Events," JAMA 274 (1): 42 (1995).

[6] Bates, "Incidence," 31.

[7] Bates, "Incidence," 29.

[8] Bates, "Incidence," 31.

infrequency of harmful or potentially harmful errors provides little con-
solation to people whose lives are touched by such errors.

But just how much lower must the error rate go? In a 1994 *JAMA* commentary, Dr. Leape suggests that even reducing it to 0.1 percent "may
not be good enough." He supports that notion by quoting quality expert
W.E. Deming, who, writing about other high-volume activities that
demand serious precision, reportedly noted, "'if we had to live with
99.9%, we would have two unsafe plane landings per day at O'Hare
[airport], 16,000 pieces of lost mail every hour, and 32,000 bank
checks deducted from the wrong account every hour.'"[9] Considering
the millions of doses of medication administered in the United States
each year, it seems fair to assume that error rate as miniscule as 0.1
percent (one error per thousand doses) would produce error totals that
rival or exceed Deming's calculations for other industries. And given
the current error-rate estimates that researchers are generating, it seems
equally fair to argue that healthcare has a lot of work to do.

Assessing the actual death, injury, and error rates for medication use
is difficult, given the complexity of modern medical treatment and
the limitations of many studies. The 1998 *JAMA* study that pointed to
ADR as a leading cause of death, for instance, was based on meta-
analysis—a technique that involves combining data from different
studies and that the study authors, themselves, acknowledged is not
completely reliable.[10] William Kelly, PharmD, a faculty member in the
Department of Pharmacy Practice at Mercer University's School of
Pharmacy, says his research indicates the death rate may be closer to

---

[9] *Leape, "Error in Medicine," 1851.*

[10] *Lazarou, et al., 1204.*

70,000, while Dr. Leape has been quoted as suggesting that it may be closer to 50,000.[11] Although these estimates are significantly lower, both are still disturbingly high, and there is widespread agreement that ADE and ADR pose real threats to patient well-being.

The myth of infallibility

It sounds like a paradox, but a growing number of experts say that one of the best ways to address the problem of preventable ADE is to accept the fact that we cannot prevent them all. Their views are based upon two realities: First, the toxicity of many medications means there is an inherent risk in taking them. Healthcare professionals constantly weigh the risk of side effects against a drug's likely benefits, and, at times, rare reactions lead to tragedies that an individual or organization could not reasonably be expected to anticipate.

The second reality is that healthcare professionals are human; they make mistakes. Researchers say unwillingness to accept this fact, both inside and outside healthcare, creates an atmosphere that makes errors more likely and harder to prevent. For the sake of patients, the argument goes, it is important to maintain a zero-error standard. But if we blame and sanction healthcare professionals when they make an error, we discourage them from reporting mistakes. Inconsistent reporting makes it difficult to identify the patterns of occurrence necessary for developing effective strategies for prevention.

In addition to overcoming this myth of infallibility, tort reform—to insulate individuals from malpractice liability—might set the stage for more effective reporting of ADE. But while that issue is debated, many

---

[11] Denise Grady, "Study Says Thousands Die from Reaction to Medicine," The New York Times, April 15, 1998, A21.

people are looking for ways to reduce the impact of ADE, and most see potential models in other so-called "high-risk" industries.

Aviation and the human factor

The Aviation Safety Reporting System (ASRS) is one such model. Founded by the Federal Aviation Administration and NASA, the ASRS provides a channel for voluntary reporting of safety violations in aviation. Reporting of non-criminal incidents is confidential, and those who file reports are generally granted immunity from punishment for any role they played in the reported incident (for more, see Exhibit A).

Industry officials and regulators embraced this confidential, non-punitive approach to reporting after accepting the notion that, while human error might be the immediately observable reason for an incident, the "root cause" is generally a flaw in the systems governing human action. This hypothesis forms the foundation for a field of cognitive psychology known as human factors research. Experts in this field have found that there are conditions and environments in which humans are more likely to err. In many fields where errors are unacceptable, their findings have prompted the development of systems and procedures that are designed to insulate humans from error-producing situations.

In aviation, officials realized that, before they could address systemic flaws, they needed a comprehensive database of safety-related incidents that would reveal patterns of error and help them understand where their systems were breaking down. Agreeing to protect the careers and reputations of pilots, air-traffic controllers, flight attendants, mechanics, ground personnel, and others who are likely to provide

Exhibit A

NASA Aviation Safety Reporting System

Overview

The Federal Aviation Administration (FAA) and the National Aeronautics and Space Administration (NASA) established the Aviation Safety Reporting System (ASRS) in 1975. FAA provides most of the program's funding. NASA administers the program and sets its policies—in consultation with the FAA and the aviation community.

Purposes

Based in Moffett Field, California, the ASRS collects, analyzes, and responds to voluntarily submitted aviation-safety incident reports to lessen the likelihood of aviation accidents. ASRS data are used to:

- alert authorities to deficiencies and discrepancies in aviation so these issues can be addressed.
- support policy-making and planning for, and improvements within, aviation.
- strengthen the foundation of human factors safety research in aviation.

This final objective is particularly important, since it is generally conceded that over two-thirds of all aviation accidents and incidents are, at their root, the result of human-performance errors.

NASA Aviation Safety Reporting System (continued)

Reporting incentives

Pilots, air-traffic controllers, flight attendants, mechanics, ground personnel, and others involved in aviation operations submit reports to the ASRS when they are involved in, or observe, situations that compromise aviation safety. Reporting is voluntary, and ASRS holds all reports in strict confidence.

ASRS staff remove all personal and organizational names from reports for entry into the program's database. They generalize or eliminate dates, times, and related information—anything that could suggest an identity. As of 1998, more than 300,000 reports have been submitted, with no breaches of confidentiality.

The FAA offers limited immunity to reporters. The agency does not, for instance, use ASRS information against reporters in enforcement actions. The FAA also waives fines and penalties for unintentional violations of federal aviation statutes and regulations—if those violations are reported to the ASRS within ten days, and provided the reporter has not violated federal aviation regulations or the Federal Aviation Act within five years.

NASA Aviation Safety Reporting System (continued)

Report processing

Incident reports are read and analyzed by the ASRS's staff of safety analysts, which is composed entirely of pilots and air-traffic controllers. Analysts come from all sectors of the aviation industry, and most have decades of experience.

At least two analysts read each report. They identify aviation hazards and flag them for immediate action. Then the analysts diagnose the root causes for each reported event. Their observations and reports go into the ASRS database, which provides information for alerts on specific hazards. The database is also a source of information for ASRS safety publications, and it supports policy-making and research on aviation safety.

Source: Excerpted, with minor adaptation, from "Program Overview" on the ASRS website: olias.arc.nasa.gov/asrs/ASRS.html.

such information removed a potentially debilitating barrier to reporting and is generally thought to have increased the reliability of ASRS data. An increasing number of people are saying that healthcare needs to offer similar protection to people who report medication errors.

Applying systems analysis to healthcare

To support their call for applying the findings of human factors research and systems analysis to the prevention of ADE, researchers have begun identifying risk points along the medication-use continuum. This continuum can be divided into four general stages: 1) prescribing and ordering, 2) verifying and dispensing, 3) reverifying and administering, and 4) educating and monitoring (see Figure 1.1).

This four-stage process already bears many hallmarks of a system designed to prevent errors. Most notably, it includes internal checks and balances. Physicians, for instance, are expected to check the patient's chart for known allergies, possible drug interactions, and/or record of other medical conditions—all of which could affect their choice of medication. Pharmacists double-check a patient's allergy and interaction profile, and confirm that the prescribed dosage, timing, and method of administration make sense. Nurses check all that information again before administering the medication, and they ensure that the pharmacy has actually dispensed what the doctor prescribed.

At its simplest level, this system operates under the assumption that a fresh set of eyes can help protect patients—either by catching a mistake made earlier in the process or by correcting for another person's lack of understanding or poor judgment. It also reflects the healthcare industry's acknowledgment that treatment with medication is a

Figure 1.1	The medication-use continuum	

Stage	Individual(s) Involved	Actions & Responsibilities
Prescribing and Ordering	Physician*	Physician examines patient, makes diagnosis, and prescribes medication after checking patient chart for allergies and possible drug-drug interactions.
Verifying and Dispensing	Pharmacist	Pharmacist reviews and fills prescription, after checking the dose and indication, that the prescription does not duplicate an existing order, and that there is no known risk of reaction due to allergy or interaction with other drugs.
Reverifying and Administering	Nurse	Nurse receives medication, checks to ensure pharmacy dispensed right drug in proper form and dose, and, after triple-checking allergy profile, administers as ordered by physician.
Educating and Monitoring	Nurse** Pharmacist** Physician Patient	Caregiver(s) instructs patient as to indication and intended effects of medication and its proper use.

The medication-use continuum (continued)

Stage	Individual(s) Involved	Actions & Responsibilities
Educating and Monitoring *(continued)*	Nurse** Pharmacist** Physician Patient *(continued)*	Caregiver(s) listens and responds appropriately to patient comments: • "I took that drug once before, and it made me sick!" • "When I filled my last prescription the tablets were red. Why are they white now?" • "Why am I taking medicine for diabetes? I don't have diabetes." Caregiver(s) monitors patient for unintended and/or adverse effects, and to ensure patient complies with medication regimen.

*In some states, nurse practitioners and physician assistants also have the authority to prescribe medication.

**Because nurses often have the most interaction with patients in inpatient settings, they tend to perform monitoring and education activities in those settings. Pharmacists often play a significant role in outpatient monitoring and education. As will be discussed in the next chapter, it's thought that increasing pharmacist involvement in treatment and education across all settings could help reduce the frequency of errors and ADR.

complex undertaking, one that requires more expertise and knowledge than an individual can or should be expected to attain.

That's one reason why most United States hospitals have embraced unit-dose distribution (see Figure 1.2), a system that's based upon checks and balances and applies a division-of-labor approach to error prevention. It ensures, for instance, that pharmacists prepare medication and dispense single doses to patient-care areas, where nurses handle administration (the alternative being storage of bulk supplies on wards, where personnel who lack a pharmacist's knowledge of drugs and chemicals, who may be distracted by other duties, and whose work might not be checked, measure and compound doses). Organizational approaches to unit-dose distribution may vary slightly, but all unit-dose systems share at least four components:

1. Drugs are stored in and administered from a labeled package that contains a single dose.
2. Medications are, as much as possible, ready to administer when dispensed.
3. No more than one day's worth of drugs are stored in patient areas at one time.
4. Floor stocks of medication are limited.[1]

Charting the current system's flaws

It is become increasingly clear that, despite unit-dose distribution and the four-stage continuum outlined in Figure 1.1, too many medication errors occur. To begin creating strategies for improvement, researchers

---

[1] Neil M. Davis, Michael Cohen, et al., Medication Errors: Causes and Prevention (Huntingdon Valley, PA: Neil M. Davis Associates, 1981), 4.

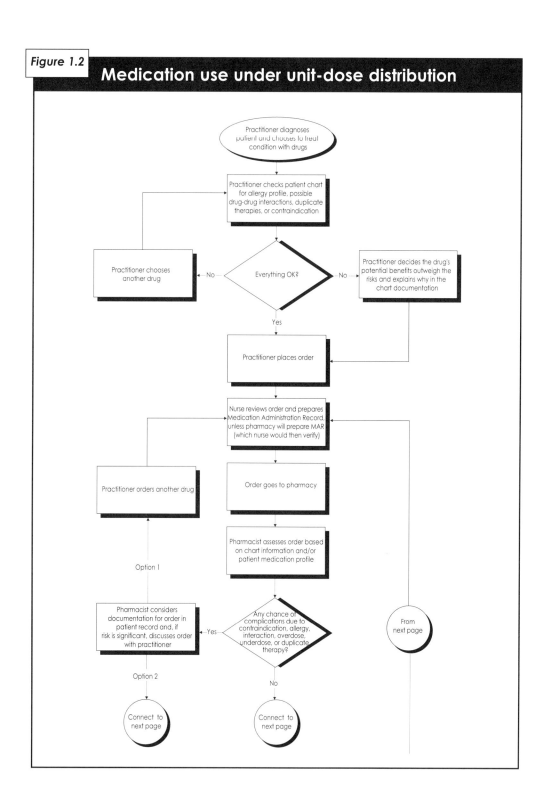

Figure 1.2

Medication use under unit-dose distribution

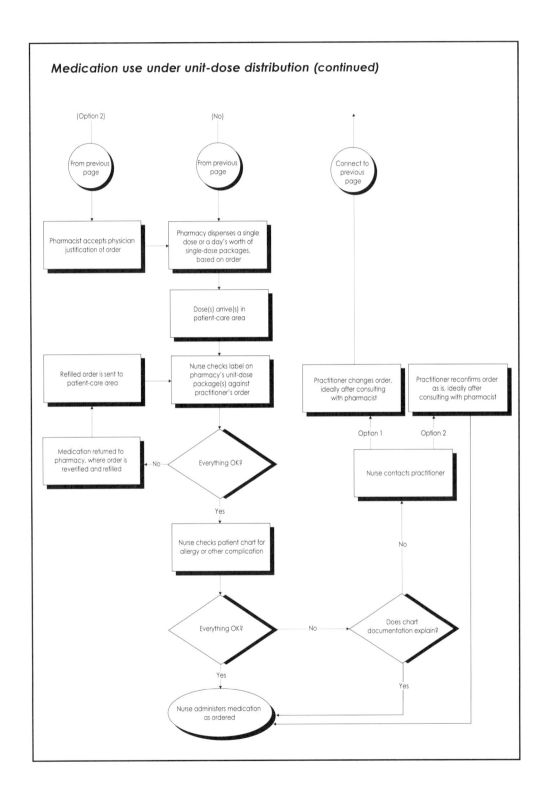

Medication use under unit-dose distribution (continued)

are searching for patterns of error that allow them to address additional risk-points along the medication-use continuum. For instance, common errors are highlighted in industry publications—like *Medication Errors: Causes and Prevention*, a landmark book by Neil Davis, and Michael Cohen. Likewise, an article by Trent Howard in the winter 1997 edition of the *Southern Journal of Hospital Pharmacy* describes several potentially fatal drug interactions (see Figure 1.3) and is indicative of ongoing efforts to provide pharmacists, physicians, and nurses with information that can prevent tragic errors.

There's no question that such lists and alerts provide valuable information. But how often is that information available at the moment a drug is being prescribed, dispensed, or administered? And, given the hectic nature of many healthcare facilities and the complexity of modern treatments, is it reasonable to expect doctors, pharmacists, and nurses to remember everything they need to know about medication? Most people agree that such an expectation is not reasonable, so researchers have begun to dig deeper, determining which errors occur most frequently, searching for the systemic root causes that underlie them, and recommending improvements designed to make it harder for the same or similar errors to keep occurring.

That was, in fact, the intent of the 1995 research led by Dr. Leape and Dr. Bates. That study, which tracked ADE across 11 units at Brigham and Women's Hospital and Massachusetts General Hospital in Boston, was one of the first to apply systems-analysis criteria to the full medication-use continuum. Over six months, the researchers identified 264 adverse events that involved a total of 334 medication errors.[12] Seventy-five percent of the ADE were the result of initial

---

[12] *Leape, "Systems Analysis," 35.*

Figure 1.3

Drugs that don't mix

This table, based on information from an article by Trent Howard in the *Southern Journal of Hospital Pharmacy*, highlights nine potentially fatal drug interactions. Many organizations disseminate such information, which can help prevent harm to patients. Nonetheless, researchers who study medication errors advocate the design of systems for avoiding these and other interactions that are less dependent on human memory and observation.

Interacting Drugs	Potential Complications
clonidine (Catapres®) & propranolol (Inderal®)	Sudden withdrawal of clonidine from combined therapy with propranolol can cause fatal rebound hypertension.
fluoxetine (Prozac®) & tranylcypromine (Parnate®)	Combining these drugs can result in a severe, sometimes deadly, condition known as central serotonin syndrome.
warfarin (Coumadin®) & oxyphenbutazone (Oxalid®)	Oxyphenbutazone can increase the anticoagulant effects of warfarin, sometimes causing fatal hemorrhaging.
digoxin (Lanoxin®) & quinidine (Quinora®)	Combination of these drugs often results in an increased plasma concentration of the glycoside, the effects of which range from GI side effects to sudden death.

Drugs that don't mix (continued)

Interacting Drugs	Potential Complications
spironolactone (Aldactone®) & potassium chloride	Combining these drugs can cause hyperkalemia, a condition that can lead to cardiac arrest and death.
theophylline (Theodur®) & ciprofloxacin (Cipro®)	Combining these drugs has been known to cause deadly seizures.
tolbutamide (Orinase®) & phenylbutazone (Azolid® and Butazolidin®)	Combination of these drugs can cause a fatal hypoglycemic response.
methotrexate (Folex®) & non-steroidal anti-inflammatory agents (NSAIDS)	Combining high doses of methotrexate in patients also taking NSAIDS can produce a deadly toxic response.
phenytoin (Dilantin®) & dopamine (Intropin®)	Concurrent use of these drugs has produced dramatic, potentially fatal, hypotension.

Source: Trent Howard, "Ten Drug Interactions Every Pharmacist Should Know," Southern Journal of Hospital Pharmacy, Winter 1997, 13-16. One interaction that Howard identifies is not noted here, because it involves a drug that is no longer on the market.

errors made during the ordering or administration stages (see Figure 1.4), prompting Leape and Bates to call for preventive efforts that emphasize these stages.[13]

---

[13] Bates, "Incidence," 33.

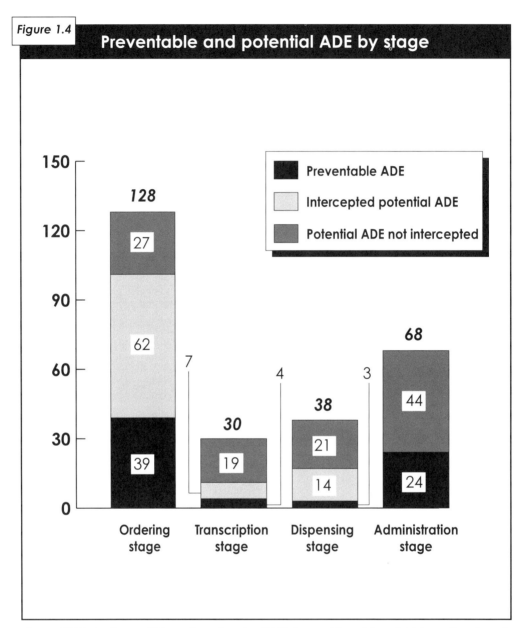

Figure 1.4

Preventable and potential ADE by stage

Legend:
- Preventable ADE
- Intercepted potential ADE
- Potential ADE not intercepted

Ordering stage: 128 (27, 62, 39)
Transcription stage: 30 (7, 19, ...) with 7
Dispensing stage: 38 (4, 21, 14) with 3
Administration stage: 68 (44, 24)

Source: "Table 6. — Stages of Primary Errors Associated With Preventable and Potential Adverse Drug Events" in David W. Bates, David J. Cullen, et al., "Incidence of Adverse Drug Events and Potential Adverse Drug Events," JAMA, 274 (1): 33 (1995).

After tallying these errors and sorting them by medication-use stage, the researchers classified and ranked them according to "proximal cause" (see Figure 1.5), which they consider the "apparent 'reason' [an] error was made"[14] but not the root cause. Say, for instance, a patient dies after a nurse administers too much potassium chloride; the proximal cause, or the most apparent reason for the patient's death, is the nurse's mistake. Traditionally in healthcare, that's as far as an inquiry into such an incident might go; the nurse would be blamed, sanctioned, and retrained. The healthcare organization might have to compensate the patient's family and would undoubtedly seek to move on—at least until the next potassium-chloride overdose.

Researchers like Kelly, Davis, Cohen, Leape, Bates, and others say that this blame-and-move-on approach makes "the next error" almost inevitable. Proximal causes, they argue, are only the most visible components of larger problems that are deeply rooted and hidden in the very systems that govern medication use. As long as those systems remain unchanged, the cycle of error can't be broken. So Leape and Bates went deeper in their study, analyzing proximal causes for the ADE they observed and identifying 16 underlying systems failures (see Figure 1.6), which they believed were ultimately to blame.

Of these 16 systems failures, the seven most frequent (which accounted for nearly 80 percent of the errors observed) all involved access to information—on either a drug or a patient.[15] Most of the other systems failures were associated with management and training issues—the

---

[14] Leape, "Systems Analysis," 36.

[15] Leape, "Systems Analysis," 41.

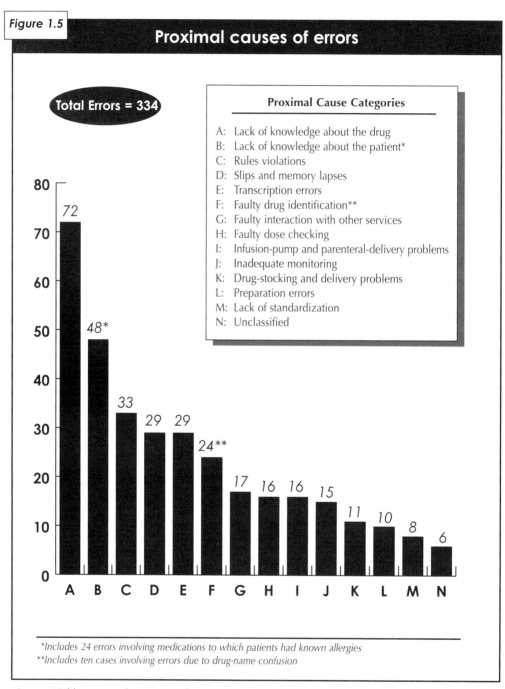

Figure 1.5

Proximal causes of errors

Total Errors = 334

Proximal Cause Categories

A: Lack of knowledge about the drug
B: Lack of knowledge about the patient*
C: Rules violations
D: Slips and memory lapses
E: Transcription errors
F: Faulty drug identification**
G: Faulty interaction with other services
H: Faulty dose checking
I: Infusion-pump and parenteral-delivery problems
J: Inadequate monitoring
K: Drug-stocking and delivery problems
L: Preparation errors
M: Lack of standardization
N: Unclassified

72 — A
48* — B
33 — C
29 — D
29 — E
24** — F
17 — G
16 — H
16 — I
15 — J
11 — K
10 — L
8 — M
6 — N

*Includes 24 errors involving medications to which patients had known allergies
**Includes ten cases involving errors due to drug-name confusion

Source: "Table 4.—Distribution Errors by Proximal Cause and Stage of Drug Ordering and Delivery," in Lucian L. Leape, David W. Bates, et al., "Systems Analysis of Adverse Drug Events," JAMA 274 (1): 39 (1995).

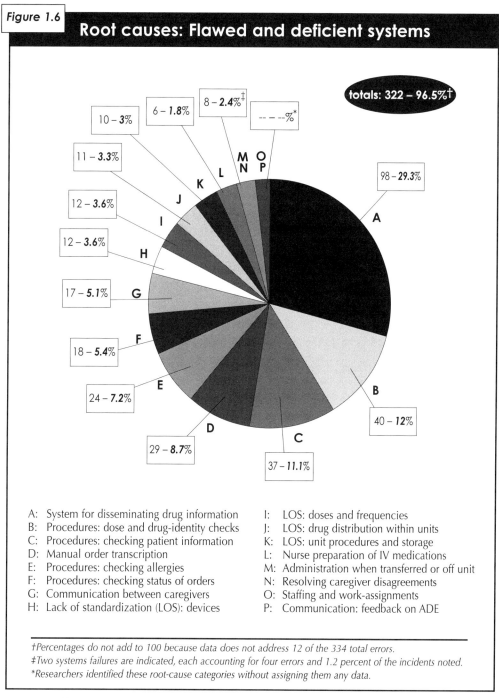

Figure 1.6

Root causes: Flawed and deficient systems

totals: 322 – 96.5%†

10 – 3%
6 – 1.8%
8 – 2.4%‡
-- -- --%*

11 – 3.3%
12 – 3.6%
12 – 3.6%
17 – 5.1%
18 – 5.4%
24 – 7.2%
29 – 8.7%
37 – 11.1%
40 – 12%
98 – 29.3%

A: System for disseminating drug information
B: Procedures: dose and drug-identity checks
C: Procedures: checking patient information
D: Manual order transcription
E: Procedures: checking allergies
F: Procedures: checking status of orders
G: Communication between caregivers
H: Lack of standardization (LOS): devices

I: LOS: doses and frequencies
J: LOS: drug distribution within units
K: LOS: unit procedures and storage
L: Nurse preparation of IV medications
M: Administration when transferred or off unit
N: Resolving caregiver disagreements
O: Staffing and work-assignments
P: Communication: feedback on ADE

†Percentages do not add to 100 because data does not address 12 of the 334 total errors.
‡Two systems failures are indicated, each accounting for four errors and 1.2 percent of the incidents noted.
*Researchers identified these root-cause categories without assigning them any data.

Source: "Table 7.—Systems Failures," in Lucian L. Leape, David W. Bates, et al., "Systems Analysis of Adverse Drug Events," JAMA 274 (1): 41 (1995).

most significant of which, they determined, involved a general lack of standardized procedures.[16]

Armed with this powerful set of common error denominators, Leape, Bates, and their colleagues were able to make specific improvement recommendations. We'll examine these recommendations, and others, in the next chapter.

---

[16] Leape, "Systems Analysis," 41.

SUGGESTED READING

Books

Bogner, MS, ed. *Human Error in Medicine* (Hillsdale, NH: Erlbaum, 1994).

Reason, James D. *Human Error* (Cambridge: Cambridge Univ. Press, 1992).

Articles

Allen, EL and KN Barker. "Fundamentals of medication error research." *Am J Hosp Pharm* 47: 555-69 (1990).

Bates, DW, DJ Cullen, N Laird, et al. "Incidence of adverse drug events and potential adverse drug events." *JAMA* 274 (1): 29-34 (1995).

Kahn, KL. "Above all do no harm: how shall we avoid errors in medicine?" *JAMA* (editorial) 274 (1): 75-6 (1995).

Lazarou, Jason, Bruce H. Pomeranz, and Paul N. Corey. "Incidence of Adverse Drug Reactions in Hospitalized Patients: A Meta-analysis of Prospective Studies." *JAMA* 279 (15): 1200-05 (1998).

Leape, Lucian L., David W. Bates, DJ Cullen, et al. "Systems Analysis of Adverse Drug Events." *JAMA* 274 (1): 35-43 (1995).

Leape, Lucian L. "Error in medicine." *JAMA* 272: 1851-7 (1994).

Leape, Lucian L., TA Brennan, N Laird, et al. "The nature of adverse events in hospitalized patients: results of the Harvard Medical Practice Study II." *N Engl J Med* 324: 377-84 (1991).

"The science of making mistakes." *Lancet* (editorial). 345: 871-2 (1995).

Applying the Systems Approach: Models for Error Prevention

The human factor

At one time or another, most people drive home from work and, upon arriving, find they have no memory of the commute. Likewise, a lot of people begin their commute planning to run an errand, only to arrive home having forgotten to stop along the way. The first instance illustrates the mind's ability to perform unconsciously tasks that are routine and familiar—even complex ones, like driving a car. The second instance, on the other hand, begins to illustrate some common human weaknesses: We're more likely to make mistakes when faced with tasks that require us to alter familiar behaviors, or that are unfamiliar. Experts in an area of cognitive psychology known as human factors research have also documented that humans tend to err when they rely heavily on memory and sensory information (like observation), and when they perform tasks that require a lot of attention or precision (for more on human factors research, see Exhibit B). In short, these researchers have found that we are generally good creative thinkers and effective problem solvers, but that we're not very detail-oriented and exact.

Errors that result from dependence upon unreliable aspects of human cognition are often insignificant. When we forget to run an errand, the

Exhibit B	Human factors research

In his book *Human Error*, human factors researcher James D. Reason argues that human actions are either automatic and governed by cognitive impulses that are triggered by familiar patterns, or deliberate and in response to unfamiliar or uncommon stimuli that call for careful decision-making. Actions in response to the first category of impulses are instinctive and are often performed unconsciously; they are the things we've done often enough to make "thought" unnecessary (like the commute discussed at the beginning of the chapter). Responses to the second type of impulses are never unconscious. Running an errand on the way home from work requires us to disengage our internal "auto-pilot" and consciously follow a different route. Driving in Britain forces Americans to pay strict attention to traffic patterns to avoid using the wrong side of the road.

Anatomy of an error

Working from that basic theory of cognition, Reason and others have begun to develop a framework for explaining how, why, and when people err. They begin by defining two categories of error— slips and mistakes:

- Slips are errors that occur during actions governed by familiar impulses. In such instances, we know or have some idea what to do, but we do it wrong or poorly.

Human factors research (continued)

- Mistakes are errors of judgment; they occur when we confront unfamiliar situations and must make a decision to act based on an inadequate supply of information. In these situations, rules and the familiar patterns of habit do not apply.

An American driver who gets in an accident in Britain because he or she does not know that the English drive on the left side of the road has, in other words, made a mistake. Someone who simply forgets the English rules of the road, or instinctively moves to the right side, has committed a slip.

According to human factors researchers, the human mind creates and stores many patterns and rules, making most functioning automatic—at least until a distraction or some other aberration from the norm disrupts the routine. The trigger might be as basic as having something else on your mind, but once the familiar patterns breakdown and you're placed in the sorts of ill-informed situations that produce mistakes, you're more likely to err. And the likelihood that you'll err increases in proportion with the complexity of the decision-making that's required, and with the length of time that you're forced to operate outside of the "routine."

The relevance of these findings to medication use is clear. Decision-making during drug treatment is often highly complex, and minor variations from case to case ensures that such decision-making is

Human factors research (continued)

rarely routine. The potential for slips and mistakes is great, particularly when caseloads are heavy. Medication-error researchers say it's critical that we begin to reduce that potential for error by designing processes that allow caregivers to avoid situations in which they're more error prone. Healthcare professionals should be allowed and encouraged, instead, they say, to focus on activities that draw on their natural cognitive strengths: creative thinking and problem solving—activities like development of diagnoses and creation of overall treatment plans and strategies.

results are rarely earth-shattering or irreversible. But when an activity is potentially dangerous—as the use of medication can be—these sorts of errors and oversights can be disastrous. That's why individuals who call for a systems-analysis approach to preventing adverse drug events (ADE) favor the development of medication-use procedures and systems that are less reliant on functions like human memory, observation, calculation, and careful attention to detail.

That's not to say they want healthcare professionals to throw caution to the wind; the vigilance of doctors, nurses, pharmacists, and others will always play an important role in ensuring the appropriate and safe use of medication. However, the current system of prescribing, ordering, dispensing, and administering medication often places the onus on individuals to avoid making the kinds of mistakes that they incline toward naturally. Systems-analysis advocates say that's foolish—particularly when more reliable alternatives exist.

Systems-analysis advocates also oppose the practice of sanctioning individuals for errors that, at their root, may be the result of systemic flaws that those individuals cannot control. They err; we sanction and cajole, say researchers. We say, "You must do a better job. You must be more careful." But we rarely take steps to improve the medication-use system in ways that help individuals "do better." That, suggest researchers, is a little like building cars without brakes and blaming individual drivers for the accidents that result. Systems-analysis advocates say everyone will be better served if we add brakes, so to speak—if we make it harder to commit an error, and more difficult for mistakes to go undetected long enough to harm a patient.

Unit-dose distribution: Just the beginning?

As discussed in the previous chapter, most people see unit-dose distribution as a step in the right direction. By ensuring that a number of
skilled people are involved in medication use, this system increases
the odds that a mistake by one person will be noticed and addressed
by another before an ADE occurs. But even unit-dose distribution
leaves many important and difficult decisions in the hands of individuals,
and it often forces those individuals to make those decisions based
on interpretation, observation, and memory. Doctors who diagnose an
illness, for instance, may choose a drug to treat it and write an order
that tells pharmacists and nurses how and when the patient should
receive that drug. Assuming the physician made the right diagnosis,
chose an appropriately indicated drug, and assigned the correct dose,
schedule of administration, and route of administration (none of which
is guaranteed, even for the best-trained doctors), what if no one checks
a patient's allergy profile? What if someone does, but misreads or overlooks a key piece of information? What if the pharmacist misreads the
doctor's handwritten prescription and dispenses the wrong drug? What
if a nurse fails to check, or misreads, the label on that improperly dispensed drug? What if the nurse confuses medications that are intended
for patients sharing the same hospital room?

Many factors and events can produce an adverse event—even though
well-trained, well-intentioned people are doing everything in their
power to prevent it. Advocates for a systems-analysis approach to prevention want to give healthcare professionals the tools and support
they need to avoid ADE whenever possible. Backed, in many cases, by
research, they have begun to offer proposals for change that may make
drug treatment safer.

Standardization: Leaving less to chance

As noted previously, research by Lucian Leape, MD, of the Harvard School of Public Health, and David Bates, MD, of Brigham and Women's Hospital in Boston, suggests that organizational efforts to standardize procedures and equipment may help reduce the likelihood of medication errors.[1] That may sound like common sense; standardization—whether it's applied to the types of equipment in use, or to the policies and procedures that govern the control and use of medication—would help ensure that medication-use processes are familiar and that people are less likely to commit errors in a familiar environment. Nonetheless, while analyzing 247 adverse drug events at Massachusetts General Hospital and Brigham and Women's Hospital, Leape and Bates found a striking lack of standardization. For example:

- One of the hospitals used eight types of infusion pump. That variety, the researchers argued, confused staff and increased the likelihood for misuse and error. The hospital has since reduced the number of devices in use.[2]

- One of the hospitals employed six different K-scales, which are used to calculate doses for potassium replacement. The variation, Bates and Leape found, made miscalculations and improper dosing more likely. The organization now uses two scales. However, Bates and Leape stressed that such inconsistency is indicative of a more general lack of standardization

---

[1] Lucian L. Leape, David W. Bates, et al. "Systems Analysis of Adverse Drug Events," JAMA 274 (1): 41 (1995).

[2] Leape, "Systems Analysis," 39.

in medication ordering at both hospitals.[3] And, in an interview Bates said that he has seen a similar lack of standardization elsewhere.

- The hospitals did not locate medication carts, order forms, or medication administration records consistently from unit to unit, creating the potential for confusion among doctors and nurses who treat patients on more than one unit.[4] In an earlier article, Leape called the inconsistent location of cardiac-resuscitation equipment on wards, "bizarre, and really quite inexcusable;"[5] his and Bates's 1995 findings suggest that such inconsistencies with regard to medication should be considered equally dangerous and unacceptable.

The promise of technology

For years, healthcare has acknowledged the potential for computers to improve quality and safety, but little progress has been made toward realizing that potential. In some cases, that's because "old-guard" professionals remain married to traditional methods. In others, the cost of developing and maintaining computer systems discourages their application. And sometimes technologies simply are not yet capable of performing as needed—although that's less often the case these days. Whatever the reason, use of technology to help ensure quality and accuracy during high-risk activities—like medication use—is less pervasive in healthcare than it is in other industries.

---

[3] Leape, "Systems Analysis," 39.

[4] Ibid.

[5] Lucian L. Leape, "Error in Medicine," JAMA 272 (23): 1856 (1994).

There are tentative indications, however, that acceptance of technology is taking root. A 1998 survey by Deloitte & Touche Consulting Group suggests that use of technology in healthcare will increase in the next few years. It appears that administrative and business applications will account for much of that increase, but just over half the healthcare CIOs who responded said that, within two years, they expect their organizations to be using hand-held computers—devices with a portability that is well-suited for clinical settings. And 14.5 percent report already using hand-held computer technology.[6]

Computerized prescribing

The Deloitte & Touche survey is just one small indicator, however. Many researchers are frustrated that there's been so little progress made in applying computer technology to the prescribing and ordering process. During an interview for this book, Dr. Neil Davis, a pharmacist who has studied medication errors for some 30 years, said that it's a national disgrace that physicians still handwrite medication orders. He estimates that the handwriting in 33 percent of those orders is poor to illegible. Computerized prescribing and ordering would, say Davis and others, eliminate the dangerous guessing game that pharmacists sometimes play when deciphering a scrawled prescription.

It promises to do much more, as well. Bates and Leape, for instance, found that nearly 80 percent of the errors noted during their study of ADE might have been prevented if healthcare professionals had access to timely information—either on the drug(s) in question or on the patient involved. The researchers argued that computers offer the most

---

[6] *Deloitte & Touche Consulting Group, "1998 Global Survey of Chief Information Executives," (New York: Deloitte & Touche Consulting Group, 1998), 33.*

reliable means for providing such information.[7] Their study also found that errors occurred most frequently at the prescribing and ordering stage.[8]

Brigham and Women's Hospital (BWH), a 700-bed facility, installed a computerized order-entry system to test Leape's and Bates's hypothesis regarding the prevention potential of computers (see Figure 2.1). The researchers monitored the results over an eight-month period and, in a follow-up study, reported that the system reduced the incidence of serious medication errors by 55 percent.[9]

The BWH system supports physician decision-making during order-entry by checking a drug's indication against the doctor's diagnosis. It also looks for allergies and drug interactions. And it determines if the order is appropriate, given the results of recent lab tests. The computer flags potential problems immediately, and it requires the doctor to address those problems before submitting the order. The doctor has the option to override the computer and enter an order unchanged, but only by entering an explanation for that override. Explanations are forwarded to the pharmacy for consideration, where the order may be challenged.

BWH's computer system also displays a menu of acceptable doses for the drug in question, and it suggests an optimal dose based on the patient's age and kidney function. Finally, it won't accept an order until the physician has chosen a dose, route of administration, and dosing

---

[7] Leape, "Systems Analysis," 41-2. and David W. Bates, David J. Cullen, et al., "Incidence of Adverse Drug Events and Potential Adverse Drug Events," JAMA 274 (1): 33 (1995).

[8] Leape, "Systems Analysis," 37.

[9] David W. Bates, Lucian L. Leape, et al. "Effect of Computerized Order Entry and a Team Intervention on Prevention of Serious Medication Errors," JAMA 280 (15): 1313 (1998).

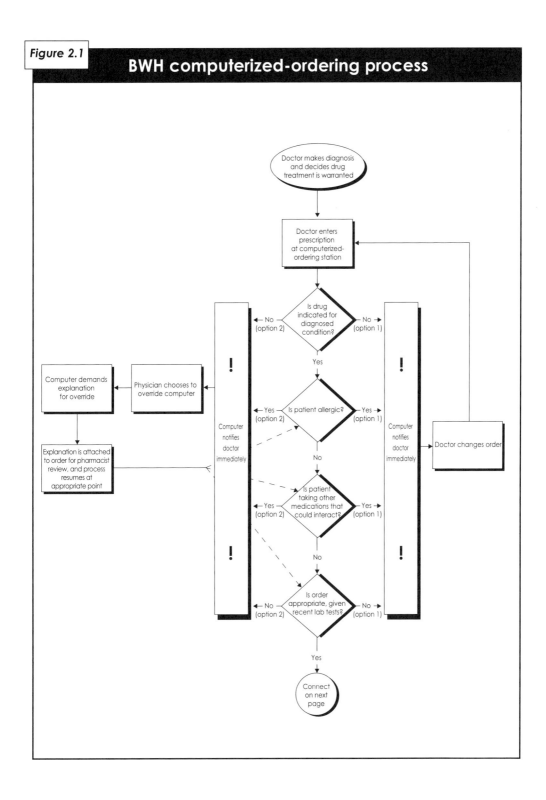

Figure 2.1

BWH computerized-ordering process

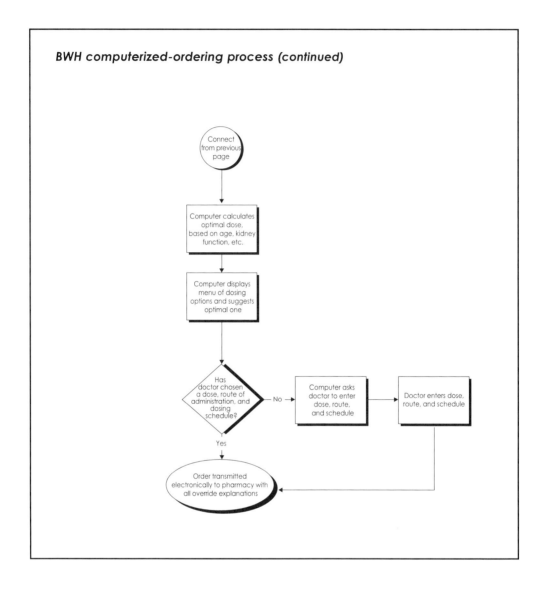

BWH computerized-ordering process (continued)

schedule. Required steps like these, known as forcing functions, are designed to make it harder for doctors to enter bad information or to leave key information off an order.

The system eliminates reliance on handwritten and verbal orders (which must be transcribed)—an arrangement that is unquestionably error-prone. It also adds another layer of checks and balances to the order-entry and order-verification processes—one that is, in all likeli-hood, more reliable; computers perform search-and-confirm activities faster and more accurately than humans and are not affected by fatigue, stress, and the distractions common to busy healthcare settings.

Bates and Leape estimate that the cost of developing and implement-ing the computerized order-entry system was $1.9 million.[10] They say it costs BWH about $500 thousand per year to maintain the system—including, according to Bates, maintenance costs for 3,500 order-entry terminals. But they believe that the system saves BWH $5–10 million each year. About $480 thousand of that estimated savings is thought to be linked directly to a reduction in medication errors (i.e., fewer costs associated with additional treatment, litigation, etc.). But Bates said that the bulk of it comes from the system's ability to notify doctors when they're ordering redundant tests, and to suggest less expensive medications than the one initially chosen. Bates and Leape acknowl-edge that their savings estimates are "crude," but they insist that their findings suggest that computerized order entry improves quality of care and could save organizations money.[11]

During a 1994 conference on ADE, Bates sat on a panel that, among other things, called for development of systems much like BWH's. The conference was planned by the American Society of Health-System Pharmacists (ASHP), the American Medical Association, and the American Nurses Association; it was funded by ASHP. The special panel made seven recommendations for preventing adverse drug events in hospitals (see Figure 2.2). Not all of the recommendations

---

[10] Bates, "Effects of Computerized Order Entry," 1315-6.

[11] Ibid.

Figure 2.2

Recommendations for preventing ADE in hospitals

1. Hospitals should establish processes in which prescribers enter medication orders directly into computer systems.

2. Hospitals should evaluate the use of machine-readable coding (e.g., bar coding) in their medication-use processes.

3. Hospitals should develop better systems for monitoring and reporting adverse drug events.

4. Hospitals should use unit-dose medication distribution and pharmacy-based intravenous admixture systems.

5. Hospitals should assign pharmacists to work in patient-care areas in direct collaboration with prescribers and those administering medications.

6. Hospitals should approach medication errors as system failures and seek system solutions to preventing them.

7. Hospitals should ensure that medication orders are routinely reviewed by a pharmacist before first doses, and should ensure that prescribers, pharmacists, nurses, and other workers seek resolution whenever there is any question of safety with respect to medication use.

Originally published in "Top-priority actions for preventing adverse drug events in hospitals," American Journal of Health-System Pharmacy 53: 747-51. ©1996 American Society of Health-System Pharmacists, Inc. All rights reserved. Reprinted with permission (R9845).

focused on applications of technology. However, applying promising technologies was clearly a priority of the panel, and computerizing the order-entry process was the group's top recommendation.[12]

---

[12] American Society of Health-System Pharmacists. "Top-priority actions for preventing adverse drug events in hospitals," American Journal of Health-System Pharmacy 53: 747–8 (1996).

Bar coding

The ASHP panel's second recommendation calls for the use of bar-coding systems to prevent errors when drugs are dispensed and administered. Dr. Davis, a proponent of bar coding, says the ideal system would monitor who administers what to whom, and when. Once the nurse has scanned her own ID badge, the patient's ID bracelet, and the bar code, the computer would immediately check that the right patient is receiving the right drug at the right time. The system would flag discrepancies, Dr. Davis adds, and alert the nurse to problems before the drug is administered. Such a system, he notes, could print regular reports about missed doses. It could also update a patient's medication administration record (MAR) automatically—thereby reducing reliance upon individuals for timely and accurate maintenance of important documentation. In addition to catching many errors before they reach the patient, bar-coding systems could also assist with development of other safety measures by tracking error trends more reliably and objectively than systems that depend on human reporting.

As with computerized ordering, a number of pilot bar-coding systems are in use nationwide. But development of this technology also has been slow—in part, say researchers and healthcare professionals, because drug manufacturers have not agreed to universal bar coding standards. By eliminating variation, such standards would allow bar coding to take place at production facilities and ensure that codes can be read by any system in use. Advocates say such consistency would encourage more widespread development and use of the technology.

David Musa, assistant director of pharmacy at the University of Wisconsin Hospital and Clinics in Madison, Wisconsin, agrees that universal standards would help facilitate broader application of bar coding. Nonetheless, the 500-bed University of Wisconsin facility, which also supports some 350,000 outpatient clinic visits each year, is piloting such technology. The facility attaches most bar codes itself—a process that's largely effective, says Musa, but probably not as reliable as manufacturer-based bar coding. He says it's not possible for pharmacies to replicate the intensive quality-assurance (QA) processes that drug manufacturers have developed to prevent mispackaging.

The University of Wisconsin's system is an off-shoot of a robotic drug-dispensing system, which the organization installed five years ago (for more on the robot, see Exhibit C, page 48). Musa says nurses at his organization have been told not to administer medications without bar codes during the pilot. Once they've scanned the bar codes that identify the drug, patient, and nurse, the system checks that a physician has, in fact, asked that the patient receive that particular drug, in that dose, at that time. The computer also offers relevant administration advice; in the case of a drug given via IV drip, for instance, the computer would tell the nurse how fast to set the drip.

As presently designed, the system does not check for possible allergic reactions or drug-drug interactions (although it apparently could be programmed to do so); a pharmacist must approve all medication orders—after checking for reactions and interactions—before orders can be recorded in the system. That arrangement, however, offers some—albeit indirect—protection against reactions and interactions: As the system is currently designed, the computer would intervene in efforts to fill any order lacking pharmacist approval, because it would find no record of the order and would assume that the nurse was administering the medication in error.

Pittsburgh-based McKesson Automated Healthcare designs and markets the technology in use at the University of Wisconsin. One of the company's marketing managers says McKesson's systems for drug administration and monitoring cost anywhere from $700 thousand to $1.2 million, depending upon the number of wards using the system and the number of hand-held units needed.

Better monitoring and communication

The third recommendation on the ASHP panel's list calls for development of better tools and mechanisms to monitor and track medication errors. Researchers have long argued that without accurate information on error frequency and trends, efforts to develop and target prevention measures are guided by little more than educated guesswork and common sense. However, developing reliable systems and processes for reporting is a complex process.

Reporting databases, like the one maintained by the Rockville, Maryland-based U.S. Pharmacopeia, generally rely on human reporting, which, says Dr. Bates, captures about one in every 20 errors and is a notoriously unreliable method for gathering statistically representative data. Fears about punitive action and damage to one's reputation discourage such reporting. But even with guarantees of confidentiality and/or immunity from sanction, the data gathered through human reporting may be spotty and partial. Many people may not realize that they, or a colleague, have erred. Those that are aware of an error may not invest the time and effort involved in filing a report, or they may not know how or where to report an incident.

Exhibit C

Robotic drug dispensing

Before the University of Wisconsin Hospital and Clinics began experimenting with bar coding during drug administration, the organization put the technology to work as part of an automated drug-dispensing system. For five years now, a robot has filled orders for about 400 of the facility's most-prescribed medications. When staff enter these medication orders into the pharmacy's computer system, the robot automatically searches storage shelves, reading bar codes until it finds the right drug. Then it doles out the amount requested and stores the dose in the patient's medication drawer, which is also labeled with a bar code.

Since dispensing medication can be monotonous, but also requires precision and careful attention to detail, it's the kind of activity that human factors research says human cognition is not well-equipped to perform. Boredom, fatigue, distractions, a lapse in attention, or an inexplicable oversight could prompt a person to mix up drugs, doses, or patient drawers. But the robot doesn't get bored or tired, can't be distracted, and won't lose focus. The robot also won't be fooled by look-a-like and sound-a-like labels. David Musa, assistant director of pharmacy at the university, says the facility's error rate during drug dispensing has improved dramatically since the robot arrived—dropping from about one error per 200 to 500 doses when pharmacy technicians handled the work to about one per ten thousand doses now.

Robotic drug dispensing (continued)

Pittsburgh-based McKesson Automated Healthcare designed the robot technology, which, according to marketing manager Heather Clayton, costs anywhere from $500 thousand to $1.5 million. The cost is generally spread over five years, and it includes all maintenance for five years. The purchase price also includes a packaging system that allows facilities to make medication containers robot-ready. Clayton said organizations can also lease the technology for five years at roughly $70 thousand per year.

McKesson performs a costs assessment of potential customers to determine if investment in a robot could save an organization money. Clayton said their customers—the smallest of which is a 46-bed hospital in Pittsburgh—usually begin to realize a return on their investment within two years. Some savings are due, she says, to a reduction in costs associated with treating and litigating medication errors, but most are related to a reduction in labor costs. Clayton says the robot normally allows organizations to eliminate or reassign six to eight full-time employees, saving $100–$200 thousand per year in the process. And some facilities, says Clayton, have saved up to an additional $150 thousand each year because the robot allowed them to reassign pharmacists to clinical settings, where they have more direct involvement in patient care, are better able to prevent medication errors, and can provide cost-savings input about dosing, drug-selection, and other key aspects of drug treatment.

Obviously, any reporting is better than nothing, but researchers are hoping to develop reporting mechanisms that are more reliable, comprehensive, and objective; here again, they see promise in technology. Brigham and Women's Hospital in Boston and LDS Hospital in Salt Lake City, Utah, are among the organizations piloting computer-based monitoring programs. These systems generally sift through treatment notes and flag error indicators—like, for instance, treatment with one drug followed by an order for an antihistamine, which may indicate an allergic reaction to the first drug. Researchers investigating prevention strategies hope that widespread use of such monitoring systems will eventually help them track error frequency and catalog errors more accurately, which would help their efforts to design safer medication-use processes.

Dr. Davis says there's another key issue associated with monitoring that tends to get little attention: communication. Organizations that gather insight on errors internally may be able to develop effective prevention policies and procedures, but the progress often stops there. Industry-wide improvement would be accelerated, Dr. Davis argues, if hospitals shared more information and learned from each other's mistakes better. Unfortunately, he says, legal agreements cut in the wake of a medication error (and the legal or public-relations crisis that often results) regularly prohibit staff from discussing an incident.

Avoiding sound-a-likes and look-a-likes

Dr. Davis has also been a leading voice on the issue of sound-a-like and look-a-like drug names. With more than ten thousand brand-name and generic drugs on the market, it's perhaps not surprising that manufacturers sometimes have trouble generating names for new drugs that aren't likely to be confused with others. However, through his Huntingdon Valley, Pennsylvania-based company, Safe Medication Practices Consulting, Inc., Dr. Davis participates in an innovative program to assist naming efforts. Here's how it works:

- Drug manufacturers with products under development forward possible names to Davis, through a New York City-based company called Wood Worldwide.

- Fifteen doctors write mock prescriptions, using the proposed brand names, and distribute the test orders to a network of pharmacists around the world.

- The pharmacists assess the safety of the drug names by noting whether, when written or spoken, those names could be confused with others.

- Davis evaluates the opinions of pharmacists and files a report on the likely safety of a proposed name.

Davis says that no name is perfectly safe, but he says "potentially dangerous" ratings for new names are rare. His program is geared, however, toward identifying those confusing and potentially dangerous names before they lead to a tragic mix-up (for tips on avoiding confusion due to sound-a-like and look-a-like drug names, see Exhibit D).

Expanding the role of pharmacists

Pharmacists have specialized knowledge and expertise that allows them to prevent many adverse drug events and to recognize the early

| Exhibit D | **Avoiding sound-a-like/look-a-like confusion** |

Researchers have flagged hundreds of sound-a-like and look-a-like drug names. Following are some tips for avoiding the confusion that these names tend to produce:

Stay informed

Dr. Davis is the editor-in-chief of *Hospital Pharmacy*, which, in 1997, printed a list of 570 pairs of look-a-like and sound-a-like drug names.[*] The list was a modified and expanded version of an earlier list that Benjamin Teplitsky, BS, and Michael Cohen, BS, published in the February 1992 edition of *Hospital Pharmacy*. Lists like this one, though a bit unwieldy, can be valuable references.

Don't scribble

Computerized ordering and prescribing systems, like those discussed earlier in this chapter, would help eliminate the biggest contributing factor to the look-a-like problem: handwritten orders. Until such technology is more widely available, however, Davis and other error-prevention researchers constantly remind doctors that cursive handwriting is the hardest to read. They recommend that doctors write prescriptions slowly, carefully, and in neat block letters. They also urge pharmacy and nursing staff to question orders

[*] *Neil M. Davis, Michael R. Cohen, and Benjamin Teplitsky, "Look-Alike and Sound-Alike Drug Names: The Problem and the Solution,"* Hospital Pharmacy *32: 1558-70 (1997).*

that are difficult to read. And they emphasize the need for hospitals to improve channels of communication among staff.

Avoid verbal orders

To avoid the problem of sound-a-like names, doctors are often urged not to give medication orders verbally. When verbal orders are necessary, however, doctors should speak slowly and clearly. Furthermore, the nurse, pharmacist, or technician who is taking the order should verify it by repeating all elements back to the doctor. Finally, transcriptionists should be made aware of the potential for mix-ups, given enough training to understand and make knowledgeable judgments about an order, and required to confirm all questionable or unclear orders with the prescribing physician.

Bypass short cuts

Abbreviating drug names and dosing information, or using potentially ambiguous symbols, can make an already confusing situation worse. It may take a few seconds longer to write out the information, but those few seconds could prevent a potentially life-threatening mistake.

signs of unexpected and unacceptable reactions to medication. Traditionally, however, pharmacists have not been given the kind of information on, or access to, individual patients that they'd need to put that knowledge to the most effective use possible. Nor have they always seized opportunities to work with patients, doctors, and nurses to improve the safety of drug treatment. Their role in medication use, says William Kelly, PharmD, has generally been to hole up in the pharmacy and "count and pour and lick and stick." Now, say Kelly and others, pharmacists must become equal and more active partners in patient care. Indeed, two of the seven recommendations put forth by the ASHP's special panel on preventing ADE deal specifically with increasing pharmacist involvement in treatment decisions.

Ideally, say Dr. Kelly and others, hospital-based pharmacists would make rounds with doctors, offering advice and input on treatment decisions that involve medication. Brigham and Women's Hospital and Massachusetts General Hospital were among the first United States hospitals to institute such procedures, launching a pilot program after the 1995 study of ADE by Bates and Leape. Dr. Bates says that in addition to accompanying doctors while they make their rounds, pharmacists spend most of the day in the hospitals' intensive-care units—where medication use can be especially heavy and risky.

Kelly, Bates, and Davis acknowledge that initiatives like these are expensive. Keeping up with medication orders in the pharmacy and tackling new patient-care responsibilities on wards generally means hiring additional pharmacy staff. Given the current emphasis on cost-cutting, hospital administrators may balk at such measures, and Bates and Davis acknowledge that smaller hospitals—or hospitals that handle fewer drug-intensive cases—may not need to go to the same lengths as a Brigham and Women's or a Massachusetts General. Bates says smaller hospitals might consider having pharmacists only make rounds on units where medication use is common or especially risky—like intensive care or oncology. Bates also says smaller hospitals might consider having pharmacists consult regularly with physicians (once a week, perhaps) rather than making rounds. Or they might have on-call pharmacists, whom physicians could page when medication-related questions and issues arise. Davis says hospitals that can't afford the ongoing expenses related to maintaining a larger pharmacy staff should think about making a one-time investment in computer technology to support decision-making.

Kelly argues, however, that the initial costs associated with maintaining a larger, more clinically active pharmacy staff are small compared to the potential savings of such initiatives. He says his research indicates that every additional dollar spent on pharmacy salaries saves up to ten dollars in costs associated with treating medication errors. Kelly wonders whether hospitals can afford not to get pharmacists onto the wards and actively involved in treatment decisions. "My profession needs to really rise to the challenge here and say, okay there is a problem," said Kelly. "Pharmacists are so well-prepared to deal with this; the problem is they're having a hard time getting out of the basement."

SUGGESTED READING

Books

Cohen, Michael. *Medication Errors: Problems and Solutions* (Huntingdon Valley, PA: Institute for Safe Medication Practices, 1998).

Articles

Bates, David W., Lucian L. Leape, David J. Cullen, et al. "Effect of Computerized Physician Order Entry and Team Intervention on Prevention of Serious Medication Errors." *JAMA* 280 (15): 1311-6 (1998).

Bates, David W., G Kuperman, and JM Teich. "Computerized physician order entry and quality of care." *Qual Manage Health Care* 2 (4): 18-27 (1994).

Classen, David C. "Clinical Decision Support Systems to Improve Clinical Practice and Quality of Care." *JAMA* (editorial) 280 (15): 1360-1 (1998).

Classen, David C., SL Pestonik, RS Evans, et al. "Computerized Surveillance of Adverse Drug Events in Hospital Patients." *JAMA* 266: 2847-51 (1991).

Folli, HL, RL Poole,WE Benitz, et al. "Medication error prevention by clinical pharmacists in two childrens' hospitals." *Pediatrics* 79: 718-22 (1987).

Leape, Lucian L., David D. Woods, Martin J. Hatlie, Kenneth W. Kizer, Steven A. Schroeder, and George D. Lundberg, "Promoting Patient Safety by Preventing Medical Error." *JAMA* 280 (16): 1444-7 (1998).

Raschke, RA, B Gollihare, TA Wunderlich, et al. "A Computer Alert System to Prevent Injury From Adverse Drug Events." *JAMA* 280 (15): 1317-20 (1998).

Performing a Root-Cause Analysis

When the best-laid plans fail

Healthcare organizations have begun to acknowledge the core idea of human factors research: Errors happen. Despite the best-laid plans for prevention and the careful vigilance of well-trained, committed individuals, medication errors, and adverse drug events are a fact of life in modern medicine. The death of a well-known journalist—who, in late-1994, received a four-fold overdose of chemotherapy at Boston's Dana Farber Cancer Institute—provides a poignant example. The tragedy received wide coverage in the mainstream media and led to aggressive reform at Dana Farber. Less than three years later, though, a writer for *The New York Times* recounted attending a meeting at the hospital where doctors learned of another chemotherapy overdose.[1] No system is fail-safe.

But neither should we view any system as being fail-safe enough. When medication errors and adverse drug reactions occur, and when a patient dies or is seriously injured as a result, nothing will reverse the effects or ease the pain of everyone involved. But much can be done to prevent others from having to live with the same pain. Proactive application of continuous quality improvement (CQI) and reactive

---

[1] Lisa Belkin, "How Can We Save the Next Victim?" The New York Times Magazine, June 15, 1997, 32-33.

root-cause analysis can address flaws and other potential sources of error within existing medication-use procedures—protecting patients by making organizations less error-prone.

This chapter focuses on root-cause analysis—not necessarily to endorse reactive assessment; indeed, it is generally more productive for organizations to use proactive CQI to address medication-safety before a tragedy occurs (see Exhibit E, page 60). But, the Joint Commission on Accreditation of Healthcare Organizations (JCAHO) requires organizations to perform root-cause analyses following some adverse events, and this chapter is designed to help organizations meet that requirement. Still, it's worth noting that the steps and processes discussed in a reactive context here can also be used proactively.

Sentinel events, root-cause analysis, and the JCAHO

1995 was a difficult year for healthcare. But it may also be remembered as a revolutionary year. A string of tragic incidents received significant coverage in mainstream media, prompting questions about the quality of healthcare in the United States. Whether errors and other adverse events happened more frequently that year—and, more importantly, whether any increase signaled an overall decline in the quality of care—remains an open question. But the perception that something was seriously wrong led organizations, like the JCAHO, to turn to systems-analysis experts for help (see Chapters 1 and 2 for more on systems analysis).

In the fall of 1995, the JCAHO and the Annenberg Center for Health Sciences began planning a national conference to examine errors in healthcare. That conference convened in October 1996, with logistical and financial help from the American Association for the Advancement

of Science, the American Medical Association, and other non-profit
and for-profit organizations. It was a powerful coalition that hoped to
advance a new agenda for error prevention in healthcare.

Also in 1996, the JCAHO further demonstrated that its stance on error
prevention was evolving when it introduced a policy to govern responses
to "sentinel events." A sentinel is a sentry, one who sounds the alarm at
signs of trouble, and the JCAHO's classification is meant to denote incidents that require quick investigation and decisive action (see Figure 3.1).

Figure 3.1

Reportable sentinel events

- An event that causes death or major, permanent loss of function and is not related to the natural course of a patient's illness
  or condition

- A patient suicide in a setting where that patient receives
  around-the-clock care (e.g., hospitals, residential treatment
  centers, crisis stabilization centers)

- An infant abduction, or the discharge of an infant to the wrong
  family

- A rape, on facility property, of or involving a patient, employee,
  or visitor at that facility

- A hemolytic transfusion reaction involving administration
  of blood or blood products having major blood-group
  incompatibilities

- Surgery on the wrong patient or the wrong body part

Source: Joint Commission on Accreditation of Healthcare Organizations (as of September 1998).

Exhibit E	**Continuous quality improvement**

Continuous quality improvement (CQI) is a data-driven process for improving performance, which is fueled by open-minded evaluation of opportunities for change. It involves looking proactively at an organization's functions, services, and products and asking, "How can we do better?"

The data-collection and data-analysis tools and techniques for CQI resemble, and are often identical to, those used during quality-assurance (QA) evaluations. In fact, the terms CQI and QA are sometimes used interchangeably. They are, however, different processes. QA involves retrospective identification of performance defects. It assumes that some amount of error or imperfection is inevitable and, therefore, acceptable; QA is designed to ensure that the error rates stay within acceptable parameters. CQI, on the other hand, involves ongoing, proactive assessment; it embraces, at least in principle, a zero-tolerance policy with regard to error and imper-fection. Embracing CQI means welcoming change and establishing a culture that encourages change. It means accepting the notion that processes and products can always be improved, and that each error, defect, complaint, or inefficiency—no matter how small—represents an opportunity for improvement.

Root-cause analysis is more closely associated with QA, combining reactive assessment with development of improvement initiatives designed to prevent recurrences. It may allow organizations to target

Continuous quality improvement (continued)

improvement initiatives more effectively (or more cost-effectively) by focusing on actual problems instead of potential ones. However, root-cause analysis is, by definition, performed after an adverse incident occurs, and, in healthcare, such incidents may involve death or serious injury.

Complex aspects of medical treatment, like medication use, may never be completely error-free. Therefore, it is important that healthcare organizations embrace and perform root-cause analyses. But it is also crucial that they commit resources to proactive assessment and prevention activities.

The JCAHO's official definition of sentinel event—"an unexpected occurrence or variation involving death or serious physical or psychological injury, or the risk thereof"[2]—applies to medication errors. In fact, JCAHO officials have acknowledged medication errors as a leading cause of sentinel events—and possibly *the* leading cause (see Exhibit F, page 64), though unreliable reporting of medication errors makes it hard to say for sure.

When a sentinel event occurs, the JCAHO asks that an organization report it. It also expects the organization to complete a root-cause analysis—an investigation into the underlying cause(s) of the event—that JCAHO officials deem thorough and credible (see Exhibit G, page 68). Finally, the JCAHO expects the facility to develop a plan for addressing the root cause(s) and improving their systems.[3] Ideally, the JCAHO would like organizations to submit the results of root-cause analyses to a JCAHO database that tracks sentinel-event patterns and generates best-practice information regarding prevention. However, many organizations have shied away from sharing their analyses for liability reasons (see Exhibit H, page 72).

It's not surprising that the JCAHO is concerned about incidents that harm patients or that put patients at risk; its accreditation requirements

---

[2] *Joint Commission on Accreditation of Healthcare Organizations,* Sentinel Events: Evaluating Cause and Planning Improvement *(Oakbrook Terrace, IL: JCAHO, 1998), 7.*

[3] *As this book went to press, the JCAHO's policy on sentinel events was evolving. As of late 1998, it encourages organizations to report sentinel events no more than five days after becoming aware of them. It requires organizations to complete a root-cause analysis and an action plan for improvements within 45 days of reporting. If that initial root-cause analysis is rejected, organizations have 15 days to amend it. Organizations that do not complete an acceptable root-cause analysis in time go on "accreditation watch." That designation indicates publicly that a sentinel event occurred at the organization, that the organization failed to complete an acceptable root-cause analysis in the time allotted, and that it is supposed to be working with the JCAHO to do so. Organizations placed on accreditation watch have 15 days to complete an acceptable root-cause analysis or they may lose their accreditation.*

and surveys have long been designed to protect patients (for more on JCAHO surveys, see Chapter 5). The JCAHO's stance on sentinel events is important, however, because it marks the first significant, enforceable effort within healthcare to institutionalize a systems-analysis approach to preventing errors and adverse outcomes, and many healthcare providers view the JCAHO's requirements, at least in principle, as an important step toward safer medication use.

Organizing a root-cause analysis

In the immediate aftermath of an adverse drug event (ADE), a medication error, or a potential medication error/ADE (a near miss), an organization's first priority must be to protect the short-term safety of patients by identifying and eliminating sources of imminent risk. If, for instance, a hospitalized patient has been given the wrong drug, the entire nursing staff should be alerted and reminded to verify all orders before administering drugs. In addition, the hospital staff needs to look for evidence that suggests other patients may face immediate danger. Did a doctor confuse patient names while writing a series of prescriptions? Has a pharmacist or pharmacy technician mislabeled a series of doses? Once hospital officials are confident that no other patients are at risk, they can begin using root-cause analysis to develop longer-term preventive strategies.

Assembling a team

Assigning a team of qualified people to investigate an incident is the first step in performing a root-cause analysis. The most effective teams are interdisciplinary and include individuals who, as a group, are familiar with each aspect of the process under investigation. Many organizations have a permanent team or department to oversee quality

Medication errors: A leading cause of sentinel events

The reporting aspects of the JCAHO's sentinel event policy have proven legally controversial; many healthcare organizations fear that the JCAHO will not be able to safeguard the confidentiality of reported information (see Exhibit H). Once those issues have been addressed, however, the program could play a significant role in efforts to prevent medication errors and adverse drug events. In addition to requiring root-cause analyses—an approach shown to be effective for investigating performance variation and for designing improvements—the JCAHO's sentinel event policy establishes another channel for reporting adverse incidents.

Modeled in some ways after the Aviation Safety Reporting System (see Chapter 1, Exhibit A), the JCAHO's voluntary self-reporting system is, according to officials, designed to be a protected reporting venue that helps to prevent sentinel events by revealing industry-wide patterns of performance variation. To ensure that reports remain protected, the JCAHO strips them of all information that could identify patients or providers, before recording them in a sentinel-event database. Based on information from the data-base, the JCAHO publishes "Sentinel Event Alerts," a newsletter that highlights sentinel-event risks and recommends prevention strategies.

During the database's first year of operation, 1996, medication errors emerged as the leading cause of sentinel events, accounting

Medication errors: A leading cause of sentinel events (continued)

for 39 of the 194 reported incidents. Eight of those 39 incidents involved fatal doses of potassium chloride. Since it was still fairly common for facilities to store concentrated potassium chloride on wards, the JCAHO published an alert encouraging organizations to begin moving those stocks to their pharmacies.

As this book went to press, the JCAHO had received reports of more than 300 sentinel events, and patient suicides had overtaken medication errors as the most frequently reported event. However, Dr. Rick Croteau, executive director for strategic initiatives at the JCAHO, said that, if medication errors could be tracked more reliably, he believes they would rank overwhelmingly as the leading cause of sentinel events.

improvement, and these entities may provide the foundation for an effective root-cause analysis team. But this core group should be adjusted, as necessary, to ensure that team members have an appropriate mix of skills and expertise. For instance, the JCAHO recommends that teams investigating a medication error "include representatives from pharmacy, nursing, medicine, administration, and information technology or management."[4]

Once the team is assembled, choose a facilitator to coordinate the root-cause analysis. This person, who will serve as project director and as the team's liaison to senior management, must have decision-making authority within the overall organization and, ideally, should have experience with root-cause analyses and/or quality improvement. (An experienced member of the quality-improvement or risk-management department might be a good choice.) Because the facilitator must serve as a resource and guide for other team members, he or she must remain objective throughout the investigation and should not have a personal stake in its outcome. The facilitator must also avoid becoming too distracted by the details of an investigation, focusing, instead, on motivating and managing team members, keeping the overall process on track, and encouraging promising avenues of analysis.

Making teams and analysis effective

Ironically, one way to spur more comprehensive analysis of a process is to encourage people to question and explore aspects of it that lie outside their areas of expertise. People who are familiar with a process may fail to examine basic functions or to ask basic questions—either

---

[4] *Joint Commission on Accreditation of Healthcare Organizations,* Sentinel Events: Evaluating Cause and Planning Improvement (*Oakbrook Terrace, IL: JCAHO, 1998*), 66.

because they take those functions for granted or because they're afraid that asking such questions will make them seem less expert. During a root-cause analysis, however, no question is too simplistic. Effective inquiries dig down to the elementary levels of a process—where adjustments can produce dramatic, system-wide change because they affect all subsequent events and actions in the process. It's often non-experts who push an examination to this "lowest-common–denominator" level. When an expert says, "That's how we've always done things," non-experts may be more inclined to ask, "Why?" The team facilitator must invite such questioning and cultivate an atmosphere that encourages honest responses and open-minded examination—not defensive posturing or resistance.

It's also important to eliminate hierarchy from root-cause analysis teams; otherwise, members with less organizational authority may shy away from speaking their mind or asking tough questions. It is the facilitator's job, with backing from senior management, to enforce the non-hierarchical nature of the team and to encourage a frank exchange of ideas and observations. Team members may have different levels of seniority within the overall organization, but while they serve on a root-cause analysis team, no members can be seen as wielding more authority than others.

Senior managers must support and endorse the root-cause analysis process—even if they are not directly involved in it. They must ensure that team members have the time and resources needed to complete their analysis effectively, that the team has the authority to implement change initiatives, and that it is held accountable for its work. It may help focus and motivate team members if they meet with senior management at the beginning of the process to discuss goals and

Exhibit G

What makes a root-cause analysis thorough and credible?

Officials at the JCAHO consider a number of criteria when determining whether to accept a root-cause analysis as thorough and credible. According to Dr. Rick Croteau, MD, executive director for strategic initiatives at the JCAHO, these criteria address five key issues: 1) Do the people who completed the root-cause analysis have first-hand knowledge of the incident and/or the processes involved in that incident? 2) Does an organization's leadership back and support the investigation's findings? 3) Do the findings identify systemic defects rather than blaming human error or individuals? 4) Is the analysis consistent (i.e., do some parts of the report contradict or raise questions about others)? 5) Does the investigation include a review of relevant literature—to ensure that an organization draws on lessons learned elsewhere?

The JCAHO's book on sentinel events lists even more specific expectations and criteria,* which are paraphrased below:

A thorough root-cause analysis...	A credible root-cause analysis...
• identifies proximate causes (late-stage variations and related process(es) and systems;	• involves people closely associated with all aspects of the systems and processes under review;

---

* *Joint Commission on Accreditation of Healthcare Organizations,* Sentinel Events: Evaluating Cause and Planning Improvement *(Oakbrook Terrace, IL: JCAHO, 1998), 74, 77.*

What makes a root-cause analysis thorough and credible? (continued)

A thorough root-cause analysis...	A credible root-cause analysis...
• analyzes related systems and processes; • identifies underlying or systemic cause(s) of the proximate cause(s) and explains their potential role in the event; • identifies improvement opportunities or offers a defensible argument that none exist; • outlines a plan to address improvement opportunities or provides a rationale for not addressing opportunities; • explains, when improvement plans are justified: 1) who will implement; 2) when implementation will occur; and 3) methods for measuring results.	• receives support, authorization, and encouragement from senior leadership; • presents analysis that is internally consistent and conclusions that all team members endorse; • considers all relevant literature; • is disseminated to all who can benefit from its findings; • identifies systemic defects that are (or may be) linked to multiple adverse events.

objectives, and at the end to present findings and recommendations. Too many meetings could needlessly delay the analysis process, though; the facilitator should serve as the primary link with senior management during the root-cause analysis, updating management on the team's progress and communicating management feedback to the team.

Conducting a root-cause analysis

The root-cause analysis process is based on two assumptions: first, that a sentinel or adverse event is usually the end-result of a chain reaction of other events set in motion by the underlying defect(s) in a system, and, second, that the best way to prevent the recurrence of such an incident is by addressing the underlying defect(s). Conducting a root-cause analysis, therefore, means identifying each link in the chain of events leading up to a sentinel event until you find and correct the defect(s)—or the root cause(s)—that started the chain reaction.

Beginning your analysis

A root-cause analysis team should begin its work by defining, as specifically as possible, the event under investigation. What happened? In the case of an overdose death, for example, the team might begin with an event definition that's as basic as: A patient died of a drug overdose.

However, an overly general definition (like the one above) may not be very useful. At this phase of the root-cause analysis, teams need to identify as many likely avenues of investigation as possible, and the more details they consider, the more numerous, specific, and targeted their leads will be.

Based on the hypothetical definition above, for instance, the team that's investigating the overdose cannot realistically eliminate any possible causal factors, which means members might waste a lot of time looking at aspects of the medication-use system that aren't terribly relevant. At the same time, however, the general definition doesn't point to many specific possible causes either. It points to everything and nothing, so to speak. To improve both the focus and the reach of its investigation, therefore, the team needs to expand its initial definition—adding details about the patient, the patient's condition, the drug involved, and the overdose. For instance, a better event definition might be: A ten-month-old male patient with leukemia died after receiving a ten-fold overdose of cytarabine, a chemotherapy drug administered via IV drip.

The new definition points to potential avenues of investigation, while helping to eliminate others. For instance, noting the patient's age and diagnosis, a team could determine whether the physician's choice of medication had anything to do with the death. The fact that it was a ten-fold overdose could suggest that the physician misplaced the decimal point on his or her order, or that the pharmacist misread the order—prompting an analysis of drug-ordering and order-verification procedures. The fact that a chemotherapy drug was involved might prompt a review of policies and procedures governing chemotherapy treatment. The fact that the drug was administered via IV drip might signal a need to examine policies, procedures, and equipment related to dispensing and administering drugs intended for that route of administration. It might also prompt examination of manufacturing issues and procedures that could increase the chances of an overdose (e.g., Is the drug distributed in ten-dose bags that might be mistaken for unit-dose containers, producing a ten-fold overdose?). Working from a

Exhibit H

To report or not to report?

Most organizations and individuals in healthcare agree that it's important to study sentinel events and to develop initiatives for preventing their recurrence. As this book went to print, however, many were questioning the wisdom of reporting a sentinel event to the JCAHO. The American Hospital Association, the Association of American Medical Colleges, and the American Society for Healthcare Risk Management, for instance, all worry that root-cause analyses may contain sensitive information that providers can legally protect, but that the JCAHO might be forced to reveal.

At issue is whether the information in root-cause analysis documents, once it has been turned over to the JCAHO, can be protected during the discovery phase of a lawsuit. Federal law protects information shared via some peer-review channels—as do laws in many states. But many states do not protect information that is shared with the JCAHO.

The JCAHO, which is based in Oakbrook Terrace, Illinois, says Illinois law protects such communications, and JCAHO officials have said that the JCAHO will not disclose information from sentinel-event reports to third parties—even going to court, if necessary, to defend the confidentiality of this information. But because it's not clear whether other states will recognize Illinois law, the issue remains controversial, and the JCAHO has been considering options.

It's been suggested that information could be protected if organizations don't send information to the JCAHO, but rather have a JCAHO surveyor come on-site to review root-cause analyses. But some healthcare attorneys aren't so sure.

To report or not to report? (continued)

"On-site review can give organizations confidence that their documents aren't floating about," said Susan Lapenta, an attorney with Pittsburgh-based Horty, Springer & Mattern. "But in terms of whether they're entitled to confidentiality or privilege under state law, [that's] going to depend on the state statute."

The JCAHO has also developed a plan to let organizations that meet certain criteria to report events verbally. By keeping conversations general—that is, limited to an organization's general policies for responding to adverse events and performing root-cause analysis—and eliminating any chance of creating a discoverable paper trail, commission officials hope to overcome liability concerns. However, if this reporting option becomes the method of choice, it could undermine the JCAHO's goal of establishing a database of information on sentinel events for use in identifying possible industry-wide improvement initiatives.

Healthcare organizations were cautiously optimistic about the concept of verbal reporting—though most may still consult with legal counsel before doing so. Regardless of whether they report, JCAHO officials, many hospitals, and attorney Lapenta all agree that worries about reporting should not prevent hospitals from performing a root-cause analysis.

"The organization should have procedures in place so that a root-cause analysis can be done immediately if an event occurs," Lapenta said.

Source: Opus Communications, "Reaction to Joint Commission sentinel event policy," Sentinel events and root-cause analysis: A guide to best practices *(Briefings on JCAHO special report), July 1998, 3-5.*

less-specific definition, a team might eventually identify similar avenues of investigation, but the faster root-cause analysis moves in productive directions, the faster it's going to generate meaningful improvement.

Identifying late-stage variations (proximate causes)

If event definitions help identify possible avenues of investigation, these avenues generally lead to proximate causes—that is, the actions and events that are closest in time or proximity to the sentinel event. However, the term "proximate cause" is legally charged and, in the context of root-cause analysis, controversial. In legal circles, the label "proximate cause" assigns a degree of culpability, or blame, to an action or event; it suggests liability. In the context of root-cause analysis, however, proximate causes are viewed as one link in the overall chain of events that led to an adverse outcome. They contribute to that outcome, but are caused by more-deeply imbedded systemic defects. Because of the legal implications associated with the term "proximate cause," however, attorneys often counsel organizations and caregivers to avoid the term.

This book will use the phrase "late-stage variation" as a replacement for "proximate cause." The word "variation" carries fewer connotations of blame than the word "cause" does. Also, since this designation emphasizes that such events happen in the late stages of the chain of events that produce an adverse outcome, it reinforces the notion that investigations should not end with late-stage variations.

Having used their detailed event definition to identify promising avenues of investigation (likely late-stage variations), therefore, team members must next determine which of these potential late-stage variations actually contributed to the adverse event in question. In other words, their line of questioning must shift from, "How *might* this have happened?" to "How *did* it happen?" Some answers at this stage will be more obvious than others; in the overdose example above, for instance, it seems fairly clear that someone (probably a nurse) administered the overdose. In addition, a physician may have inadvertently ordered the overdose, and/or someone in the pharmacy may have mistakenly dispensed the wrong dose. Failure, in later stages of the medication-use process, to spot an earlier error would also qualify as a late-stage variation (e.g., the pharmacy's failure to note or question the dose on the physician's order, or the nurse's failure to check or question the pharmacy's work).

The team's goals, at this point in the investigation, should be to identify as many contributing late-stage variations as possible and to avoid narrowing the scope of the investigation too quickly. It's important for team members to remain patient and committed to these goals. They may face a lot of external pressure to "get to the bottom" of whatever happened—especially if a patient died or was seriously injured. The impulse to focus on the most obvious late-stage variation(s), to trace backward from there to root cause(s), and to take quick, decisive action, will be strong. However, narrowing the investigation too quickly may mean that the team overlooks important root causes— systemic defects that could eventually lead to another tragedy.

Evidence of human error, if it was a factor in the event under investigation, is likely to emerge at this stage—which is another reason why teams need to proceed carefully and tactfully as they consider late-stage variations. Careers and reputations could be at stake, and human factors research has shown that organizations often accomplish little by blaming or reprimanding individuals who have erred. Punishment may be necessary if someone is found to have knowingly violated policies and laws, but, even in these instances, the search for systemic defects should continue. (For example, a root-cause analysis team might want to determine how an individual could subvert the system and/or purposely harm a patient.)

Addressing intermediate-level issues

Investigations may turn up problems and defects in a system that are not root causes, but that still require action. For instance: What if an investigation reveals that an employee, who was involved in an adverse event, lacks the proper training and/or falsified his or her credentials? The root cause of the incident may lie buried in the organization's hiring or credentialing policies. But even before an examination of those policies is complete, the root-cause analysis team should have the unqualified person removed from duty and, depending on the situation, might recommend a staff-wide review of credentials.

Any number of situations could arise calling for such intermediate-level action, and it's important for teams to recognize and address them. But it's equally important for teams to recognize that their work does not end there. Addressing intermediate-level issues is much like trying to patch a leaking roof: it provides temporary relief, at best. If organizations stop short of addressing the root causes of an adverse event, they may soon find themselves organizing another team to investigate a similar incident.

Identifying root causes

After teams identify late-stage variations, and as they are addressing intermediate-level issues, they must continue to peel away the causal layers of an adverse event until they've uncovered the systemic defect(s) that launched the chain reaction of contributing factors. This is not a simple process, but it is relatively predictable. Healthcare organizations are finding that most root causes lie imbedded in a relatively small number of basic functions and processes that govern organizational and individual operations—like employee training and education, operating policies and procedures, work environment, equipment, and communications. Determining precisely where the defects lie in these basic functions and processes may sound like a relatively simple process, but it is not. Teams must ask one basic question—"Why did that happen?"—over and over, until members can no longer generate answers that seem reasonable or relevant.

Consider again, for instance, the hypothetical case of an overdose death: In reviewing the patient's chart, the root-cause analysis team may realize that a physician actually ordered the fatal dose. That's a key late-stage variation and an important finding, but it's probably not the root cause of the overdose. Why did the physician submit that order? Was he or she unfamiliar with the drug? Was the doctor aware of acceptable dosing levels but, for whatever reason, did he or she prescribe the wrong dose? (e.g., Did the physician intend to write .09 milligrams, but accidentally write 0.9 milligrams?) Why didn't anyone notice or question the mistake? Did someone try to question it and get rebuffed? Did their query fail to reach someone who could resolve the issue? The list of questions that teams must ask in response to an adverse event is usually long, and each time the resulting answers identify another point of failure within a system, the team must ask the key question again: "Why did that happen?"

During an interview with the physician, for instance, the team may learn that the physician was, in fact, not very familiar with the drug that killed the patient. That's a troubling realization. Could other physicians at the organization be equally ill-informed? The team might, at this point, attempt to assess how much physicians know about the drugs they're prescribing. It might also call for training initiatives and stronger policies to govern medication orders. But, as important as these steps are, they address intermediate issues—not root causes. And, as was discussed above, steps taken to address intermediate issues cannot be viewed as the end of the investigative process. Why was the physician unfamiliar with the drug that killed the patient? And, more importantly, was that information readily available when the doctor needed it?

With thousands of drugs on the market, it's probably not reasonable to expect physicians to be completely familiar with every one; so simply urging doctors to become better informed or to be more careful is unlikely to prevent similar occurrences in the future. The root issue in this case may not be lack of knowledge; rather, it's probably lack of access to information. Doctors should learn everything they can about the drugs they prescribe, but it's an organization's responsibility to ensure that, when necessary, doctors can access the information they don't have in a quick, timely, and reliable fashion. That may mean installing a computerized order-entry system that provides relevant information as a drug is being ordered (see Chapter 2 for more on such systems). Or, it may involve compiling information on the most toxic drugs in an organization's formulary, improving mechanisms for accessing that information, and writing stronger, clearer policies on using those mechanisms.

Indeed, any number of initiatives might help an organization improve access to timely, reliable information—just as any number of initiatives might help organizations address the root cause(s) of other adverse events. For the purposes of this book, the specifics of the hypothetical overdose and the preventive strategies just discussed are less important than the general process that was outlined for responding to such an incident. Organizations cannot afford to stop inquiries into adverse events until they, first, identify root causes and, second, develop, implement, and test improvement initiatives that are designed to address those causes (see Chapter 4). This can involve a significant commitment of time, resources, and energy, and it often requires an organization to take a long, hard look at itself and at issues that it might prefer to ignore. But only by addressing root causes can organizations disrupt patterns of error and prevent future tragedies.

The JCAHO's "Framework"

To assist organizations who are following up on sentinel events, the JCAHO developed an investigation grid. Titled "A Framework for a Root Cause Analysis and Action Plan in Response to a Sentinel Event,"[5] this document is designed to guide and prompt organizations through each stage of the root-cause analysis process—from event definition, through late-stage variations (what the JCAHO calls "proximate causes"), to intermediate issues/causes, and root causes.

No single document can address the full range of factors that may have contributed to an adverse event. Organizations should not assume that completing this grid will produce an effective root-cause analysis—or

---

[5] *To receive a copy of the "Framework," contact the JCAHO's Office of Quality Monitoring or visit the JCAHO's website at www.jcaho.org.*

that it will automatically lead to results that the JCAHO considers thorough and credible. However, because the grid identifies functions and activities that could have contributed to errors at various causal levels, and because it suggests lines of inquiry that might help teams dig deeper, it can be an effective mechanism for starting root-cause analyses and for jump-starting stalled investigations—especially for teams and organizations that don't yet have a lot of experience with root-cause analysis.

Tools to support root-cause analysis

One of the ironies of root-cause analysis is that, the deeper team members dig toward the root causes of an adverse event, the less certain their answers and evidence become. There is often a solid trail of evidence, for instance, pointing to late-stage variations; if a physician orders what amounts to an overdose, a written record of that order should exist. But any effort to determine why the physician wrote that order, requires speculation.

It's human nature to want neat, clean answers after a serious incident has occurred—not a list of possibilities. And it's often easier to point a finger at individuals, back up the charges with physical evidence, and move on. Perhaps that's one reason why organizations often dig no deeper than late-stage variations. But, by now, the argument against this "natural" response should seem clear: Before long, other people are going to make the same mistakes, other patients may get hurt, and an organization won't be any closer to understanding why. The object of root-cause analysis is not to locate blame for an incident; it's to identify what went wrong (or what probably went wrong), and to take steps to prevent similar incidents in the future. Effective root-cause analysis shifts the focus from the obvious actions of individuals, to less-obvious inner workings of the systems within which individuals act.

But even if that shift makes a certain amount of speculation unavoidable, it's important for root-cause analysis teams to find evidence and to test their hypotheses. Most teams rely on a number of tools and techniques to do so, and following is an explanation of some common tools they use and of the ways that these tools support the analysis process:

Interviews

Interviewing individuals about an adverse event is a basic information-gathering technique that's used in nearly all root-cause analyses. If a number of people were involved, differences in their accounts of the event often help teams identify issues and details that need further investigation. Interviewing everyone involved may also help the team identify which systems or functions broke down (e.g., if individuals acknowledge performing activities for which they are not trained or qualified, the team may need to examine policies governing human resources). Interviewing might also reveal inconsistent or confusing aspects of those systems (e.g., if an organization uses several K-scales—formulas for calculating potassium-chloride doses—an individual involved in an overdose might acknowledge being unsure which scale was in use). Memories fade quickly, however, so interviews should take place as soon as possible after an event.

Teams should not treat the interviews like interrogations; the purpose should be to gather factual information—not to locate blame. (Although information suggesting criminal or deliberately unethical activity should be dealt with appropriately.) When they approach individuals who were involved in an adverse event, members of a root-cause analysis team should stress the informational nature of the interview process.

It's also important to create an interview atmosphere that's not intimidating or confrontational. For instance, teams might want to avoid panel interviews—where individuals field questions from several team members at once and may feel as if they're being grilled.

Instead, the team should decide what information it needs and designate one person to conduct the interview. Furthermore, it's often effective to conduct interviews on a peer-to-peer basis (doctors interviewing doctors, nurses interviewing nurses, etc.), and to avoid having employees interviewed by people who are far more senior or more junior than they are.

Surveys

Surveys, another common information-gathering tool, are more structured vehicles for inquiry than interviews are. They involve asking people to respond, either verbally or in writing, to a series of prepared questions. Sometimes respondents generate their own answers; sometimes they're asked to choose from among several prepared responses.

Surveying can be a less-time–consuming process than interviewing, especially if root-cause analysis teams need feedback from many people. Surveys can also be more objective than interviews, because external factors—such as an interviewer's tone of voice and body language—don't influence responses. And, since each respondent answers an identical set of questions, response patterns generated by surveys are often more significant than patterns that emerge from interviews.

Indeed, surveys may help root-cause analysis teams determine whether views expressed in interviews are shared throughout an organization. (If, for instance, interviews suggest that confusion about a specific policy or procedure contributed to medication error, a survey could confirm whether that confusion is widespread.)

Flow charts

Flow charts use a standard set of symbols to document each step in a process (see Figures 3.2a and 3.2b). They indicate stopping and starting points, required actions, decision-making points, waiting periods, and needed documentation.

In the aftermath of an adverse event, they can help root-cause analysis teams identify where a system actually broke down, or where it is error-prone. Armed with that knowledge, teams can redesign the process to be more effective.

To create a flow chart, teams must first define the "boundaries" of the process in question by determining its beginning and end point. Then team members identify each step in the process—often by interviewing people who are involved—and write a description of each step in an appropriate symbol.

It's often easier to analyze the process in question if teams create two flow charts—one showing what currently happens (the actual sequence of events), and another showing what should happen (the ideal sequence of events). Comparing the two will reveal opportunities for improvement.

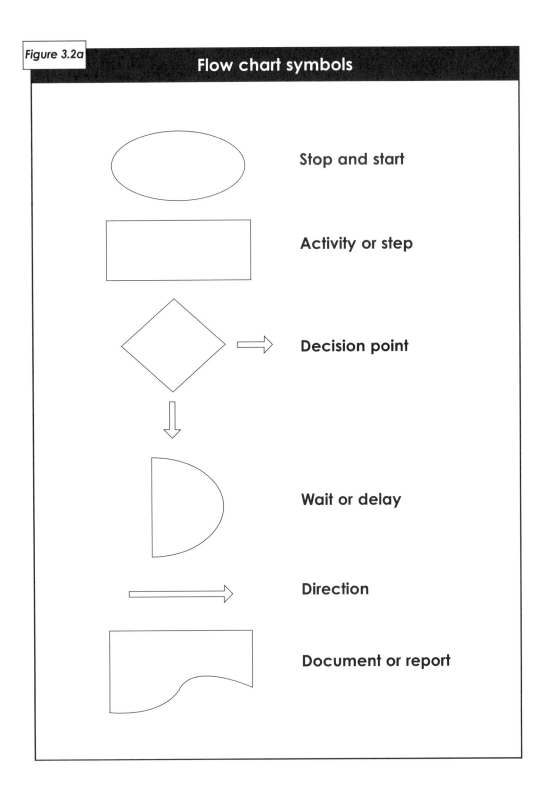

Figure 3.2a

Flow chart symbols

Stop and start

Activity or step

Decision point

Wait or delay

Direction

Document or report

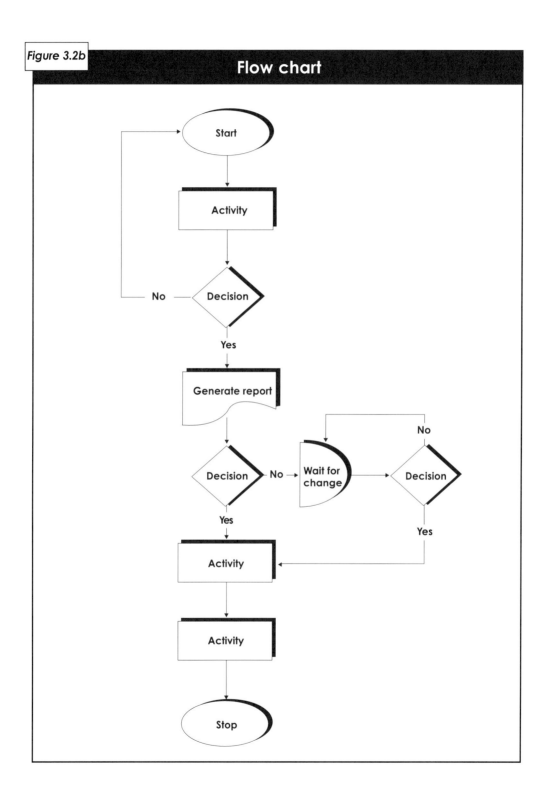

Figure 3.2b

Flow chart

Cause-and-effect diagrams

Cause-and-effect diagrams are another tool that, like flow charts, help root-cause analysis teams identify potential problem areas in a process. But, unlike a flow chart—which generally diagrams a process that is meant to produce a desired outcome—a cause-and-effect diagram begins with an unsatisfactory outcome and locates factors that contributed (or may have contributed) to that outcome. It begins, in other words, with an effect (e.g., a patient was given the wrong drug) and, by examining all the functions relevant to the process that broke down, it locates potential causes.

Cause-and-effect diagrams are sometimes called "Ishikawa diagrams"— in honor of Kaoru Ishikawa, who refined their use. Because of their appearance, they're also known as "fishbone diagrams," and building one is much like drawing a fish skeleton (see Figures 3.3a and 3.3b):

1. Team members write a definition of the problem (the effect) in a box—which is positioned at the head of the diagram with a line extending from it like a spine.

2. Team members define the core functions or causal categories that could have contributed to the effect in question, note them in boxes that are arrayed along either side of the diagram's "spine," and connect these boxes to the spine with lines that resemble rib bones. In the case of a medication error or adverse drug event, five functions are often involved: 1) equipment and materials; 2) policies and procedures; 3) work environment; 4) education and training; and 5) communication and access to information.

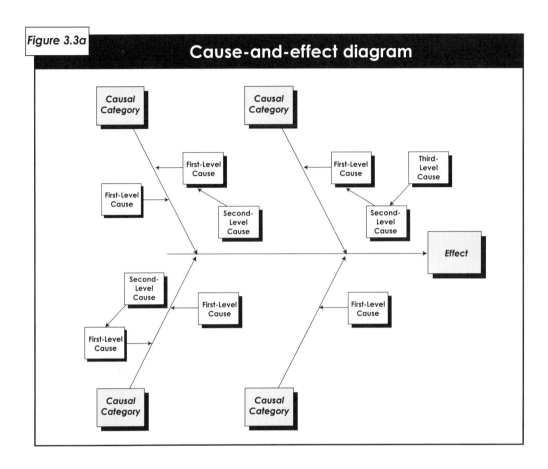

Figure 3.3a

Cause-and-effect diagram

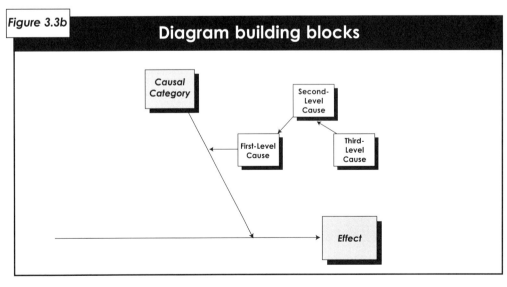

Figure 3.3b

Diagram building blocks

3. Team members identify (or brainstorm) the ways that each function contributed (or might have contributed) to the effect in question, and they write brief definitions for these potential contributing factors in boxes that are linked to the appropriate rib bone. Sometimes called possible "first-level causes," these contributing factors might also qualify as possible late-stage variations.

4. Team members identify or brainstorm potential "second-level causes" that contributed (or could have contributed) to each first-level cause. They note these "second-level causes" in boxes, with an arrow pointing to the first-level cause(s) that each produced.

5. Team members work backward from second-level causes to potential third-level causes, and so on, until they're unable to go further. The final causal level that they reach generally contains potential root causes of the effect in question.

Pareto charts

A pareto chart is a type of bar graph that displays categories of data in descending order of frequency or significance. It can help a root-cause analysis team set priorities and work efficiently because the chart identifies the most relevant and/or effective avenue for investigation or improvement (see Figure 3.4). It is a particularly useful tool for teams that have limited resources, because it helps them allocate those resources strategically.

The pareto chart is named for economist Vilfredo Pareto. He studied the distribution of wealth in 19th-century Italy and found that 80 percent of it was controlled by just 20 percent of the population. That 80–20 breakdown is often referred to as the pareto distribution, and, in

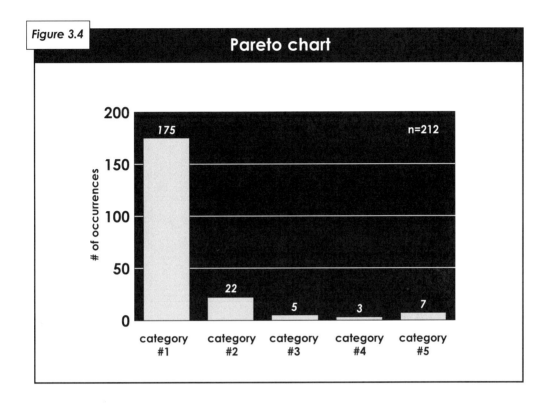

Figure 3.4

Pareto chart

the context of root-cause analysis, it has given rise to the notion that organizations can often address a great many organizational problems by addressing a small number of systemic defects (i.e., 80 percent of the problems are generated by 20 percent of the defects in a system—though the actual ratio may differ).

To use a pareto chart effectively, therefore, root-cause analysis teams must look carefully for associations between the late-stage variations, intermediate issues, and root causes they identify. If they can find a common denominator that links most of them, they may have identified a particularly significant root cause. Pareto-chart analysis won't tell teams how to address that root cause, but it will help the team focus improvement opportunities that may be particularly effective.

Research by Leape and Bates (discussed in Chapters 1 and 2) provides a good example of the potential value of pareto-chart analysis: In a study of adverse drug events at Massachusetts General Hospital and Brigham and Women's Hospital in Boston, the researchers monitored 247 adverse drug events. They traced those ADE back to 16 "systems failures," seven of which had to do with access to information—on a drug and/or a patient. Those seven systems failures accounted for nearly 80 percent of the adverse drug events that Leape and Bates monitored, which suggests that, by improving caregivers' access to information, the hospitals might drastically reduce the incidence of adverse drug events.

Decision matrices

A decision matrix is another tool that can help teams set priorities. Also known as an evaluation grid, a decision matrix is essentially a scorecard that helps teams choose objectively between several courses of action or opportunities. This tool can be particularly useful when a number of options seem equally compelling, when team members can't agree on a course of action, or when a list of possible actions/opportunities is too long to be manageable. It also ensures that each team member is involved in the decision-making process, and that each team member's input carries equal weight.

To complete this "scorecard," teams must identify their options, establish criteria for evaluating those options, and agree on a system for scoring each option based on how well it meets the requirements of a criterion (e.g., 1 = unimportant; 2 = important; 3 = very important). The options are listed down the left side of the grid, while evaluation criteria are noted along the top (see Figure 3.5a). Then each team member completes the matrix separately, totaling his or her score for

---

Figure 3.5a

Decision matrix

Rating system: 1 = unimportant 2 – important 3 = very important

Error-reduction Project

Options / Criteria	Criterion #1	Criterion #2	Criterion #3	Total	Rank
Option #1	1	1	2	4	4
Option #2	2	2	1	5	3
Option #3	3	1	3	7	2
Option #4	2	2	3	7	2
Option #5	2	2	3	7	2
Option #6	3	3	3	9	1

---

each option in the right-hand column. The totals from each individual matrix are then added together, and the option with the highest grand total is assigned top priority.

If some evaluation criteria are more significant than others, teams can assign each criterion a value or weight (e.g., 3 = low value/significance; 4 = moderate value/significance; 5 = high value/significance), which ensures that more important criteria have a greater influence on the overall scoring (see Figure 3.5b). Preliminary scores for each option are multiplied by the relevant criterion's value, producing a weighted score. The weighted scores are added to determine a weighted total. Individual weighted totals are added together, as discussed above, and the option with the highest grand total is assigned top priority.

Figure 3.5b

Decision matrix with weighted criteria

		CRITERIA					
OPPORTUNITY AREAS		Criterion #1 weight: 4	Criterion #2 weight: 5	Criterion #3 weight: 3	Criterion #4 weight: 5	Weighted-Score Total*	Rank
	Option #1	2 / 8	3 / 15	2 / 6	3 / 15	44	3
	Option #2	1 / 4	3 / 15	1 / 3	2 / 10	32	6
	Option #3	1 / 4	3 / 15	2 / 6	3 / 15	40	5
	Option #4	3 / 12	3 / 15	2 / 6	3 / 15	48	1
	Option #5	2 / 8	3 / 15	3 / 9	3 / 15	47	2
	Option #6	3 / 12	3 / 15	2 / 6	2 / 10	43	4

Scoring	Weighting
How well does this opportunity area meet the goal of this criterion?	How important is this criterion relative to the others?
1 = poorly 2 = adequately 3 = well	3 = unimportant 4 = important 5 = very important
note scores to the left of the diagonals dividing the score boxes	*weighted score = score multiplied by criterion weight

Challenging the culture of blame

The JCAHO's sentinel event policy—particularly that policy's require-ments regarding root-cause analysis—could mark an important turning point for healthcare. It could mark a shift away from blame-oriented policies and procedures toward a systems-analysis approach to error prevention. But embracing root-cause analysis and the systems-analysis approach won't be easy. Significant tort reform may be needed to make the shift as successful and as permanent as possible. Furthermore, these approaches to error investigation and prevention fly in the face of deeply entrenched mindsets that make it hard for caregivers to discuss errors, that make it difficult for organizations to look beyond the mis-takes of individuals, and that complicate efforts to get organizations to share information that may help reduce adverse-event rates throughout the industry. Nonetheless, a similar shift served high-risk industries like aviation and nuclear power well, and there's widespread agreement that, if this process continues in healthcare, the result is likely to be more effective treatment and less risk to patients.

C A S E   S T U D Y

Hospital creates infrastructure for root-cause analysis

A large hospital on the West Coast has generated internal support for, and developed a real expertise in, root-cause analysis—thanks, in large part, to strong leadership and an innovative infrastructure that supports and drives the process. According to its risk manager, who asked that the organization remain anonymous, the hospital performed about

40 root-cause analyses between October 1997 and September 1998. Some of the incidents that it investigated qualify as reportable under the JCAHO's sentinel event policy (although the hospital chose not to report them, for the legal reasons outlined in Exhibit H, page 72). However, most incidents did not meet the JCAHO's reporting criteria (see Figure 3.1, page 59)—meaning failure to investigate would not affect accreditation. The hospital often investigates non-reportable incidents though, since each incident provides opportunities to identify systemic defects that, left unchecked, might eventually lead to a patient being harmed. "We may only see the tip of the iceberg at my level," said the risk manager. "We see 1.5 million outpatients here per year, and a lot of our surgical procedures are outpatient, too, so you're looking at a whole lot of opportunities for error."

Identifying adverse events

Caregivers and departments at the hospital can report an adverse event electronically—via a site on the organization's intranet (see Figure 3.6). Or they can complete an internal reporting form designed by the risk-management department (see "Useful Forms," page 104, for a version of this form). Because voluntary reporting can be unreliable, though, the risk-management department also tracks adverse-event indicators (see Figure 3.7, page 98). Coders in the HIM department watch for these indicators, notifying the risk manager whenever one appears in a patient's record.

Advisory board makes RCA assessments

If the risk-management department learns of an incident that meets the JCAHO's criteria for reportability, it orders a root-cause analysis

Figure 3.6

Online event reporting

Description of the event: (State significant facts in chronological order)

What caused the event to occur? (State why you think this incident happened)

Date and time of the event
- Select the day: 1
- Select the month: JAN
- Select the year: 1998
- Select the nearest hour: 0100

Enter your name:

Enter your office phone number:

E-mail address:

Online event reporting (continued)

Select your department from the list: | Anesthesiology DEA |

Select the date of your report submission
- Day: | 1 |
- Month: | JAN |
- Year: | 1998 |

Departmental CI representative/chairman comments:

Is your department performing a root-cause analysis? | No |

CI Rep/chairman name: |

Enter your office phone number: |

Chairman's e-mail address: |

Select your department from the list: | Anesthesiology DEA |

Injury classification: | None/Minor |

Is this a PCE?* | Yes |

Is this a sentinel event? | Yes |

potentially compensable event

Online event reporting (continued)

(If this is a sentinel event, please submit a root-cause analysis)

Is there a patient complaint? | Yes |

Disability classification: | None/Minor |

Is a professional liability claim likely? | Yes |

Is there an opportunity for continuous improvement? | Yes |

Select the SE/PCE indicator(s) which best fit(s) the event:
Multiple items may be chosen.

Procedure performed on wrong
  patient or body part
Unexpected re-operation to repair or
  correct previous procedure
Motor weakness
Total/partial loss of limb
Loss of limb use
Blood transfusion with HIV or hepatitis
Brain damage
Sensory nerve injury
Sensory organ loss/impairment
Unplanned reproductive organ
  loss or impairment

Delayed/missed diagnosis and treatment
Unexpected death
Birth injury
Patient/visitor falls
Procedure variance
Burns or patient injuries
Operating room incidents
Material/equipment issue
AMA events
Medication incidents
Unexpected complication of
  outpatient care
Other events/incidents

Patient information:

For an inpatient, enter the admission register number: [   ]
For an outpatient, enter the outpatient chart number: [   ]

Releasability: DO NOT RELEASE. This information has been compiled and this form prepared
in contemplation of possible litigation and for assisting attorneys representing the interests
of this organization in these matters. Internal working copy permitted. Maintain internal
working documents ONLY IN DEPARTMENTAL CI FILES. DO NOT file by patient name, SSN, or
identifiers. Recommend filing by sequential log numbers.

Figure 3.7

Clinical risk indicators

- unexpected death
- transfusion with HIV- or hepatitis-contaminated blood
- brain damage
- sensory nerve injury
- loss or impairment of sensory organ
- loss or impairment of limb
- procedure performed on wrong patient or body part
- unexpected re-operation to repair or correct previous procedure
- motor weakness
- unplanned loss or impairment of reproductive organ
- birth injury

---

immediately. The risk manager reviews all non-reportable incidents and, when further investigation seems warranted, alerts the hospital's risk-management advisory board. If the board, which meets every six weeks, calls for a root-cause analysis, the department(s) involved in the incident have 30 days to comply. (The risk manager said the hospital plans to maintain its 30-day deadline—even though the JCAHO extended its deadline to 45 days in mid-1998.) The advisory board also evaluates all root-cause analysis reports and notifies analysis teams when additional analysis is needed (teams must then file an updated report before the next board meeting). To ensure that board decisions and the root-cause analysis process have the backing of hospital leadership, the board also notifies senior management of all its decisions.

Four physicians, two nurses, a claims attorney, and the risk manager sit on the risk-management advisory board. The risk manager cited three key reasons for maintaining this interdisciplinary board: First, the mix of skills and knowledge improves the board's ability to assess incidents. Second, all communication between the advisory board and root-cause analysis teams can be peer-to-peer (i.e., a physician on the board contacts physicians on a team, etc.). And, third, the peer-review nature of board decisions adds weight to the board's assessments. "Physicians know that if they get a root-cause analysis, it's not just coming from some administrator," said the risk manager.

CI representatives coordinate analysis

When the advisory board calls for a root-cause analysis, the order first goes to the continuous-improvement (CI) representative in the department where the incident occurred. That representative is responsible for coordinating the root-cause analysis process (see "Useful Forms," page 104, for an adapted version of this form). The risk manager said that about 60 percent of the CI representatives are physicians; the rest are usually senior nurses. One representative is assigned to each clinical department in the hospital.

The CI representatives are familiar with quality-improvement techniques, but the risk manager plans to have them trained to facilitate root-cause analyses, too. The risk manager hopes that the training will, first, improve the quality of departmental analysis and, second, help root-cause analysis become such an integrated part of the hospital's culture that departments will begin launching investigations without prompting from the advisory board. "Five years out, I may not have to track and trend these," the risk manager said. "I may be getting incident reports and root-cause analysis reports at the same time. That's the goal."

Careful planning sowed seeds of success

The hospital's root-cause analysis procedures and infrastructure were a full year in the making, and the risk manager worked closely with a member of senior management and a physician advisor during the planning stages. That development team also gave other key internal audiences (like nurses and other physicians) a chance to review the plan and comment. "The key to making this happen was communication and building trust with the medical staff and the nursing staff," said the risk manager. We had to stress that the focus was not to locate blame or punish individuals."

That commitment from senior management was also key. "Management and leadership have to buy into [the process]; they have to actively support it, not just say they support it," the risk manager added.

Overdose investigation tests the system

The risk manager cited a specific root-cause analysis that illustrates the potential effectiveness of the hospital's process, but also reveals the kinds of barriers that organizations often must overcome when investigating adverse events. The incident involved an infant in the pediatric intensive care unit (PICU) who received an overdose of gentamicin. Overdoses of that drug, a strong antibiotic, can cause severe hearing loss or deafness. Since infants may not exhibit obvious signs of hearing loss, overdoses in very young children can be hard to spot. According to the risk manager, this particular overdose went undetected until a doctor ordered a blood test that measured the child's gentamicin levels.

"This is a classic case," said the risk manager. "I've seen it happen several times here over the past few years. It's usually because of a communication mistake; a lot of times it's because of illegibility. It's also possible that, in mixing the drug, there's a mathematical error."

Because an overdose qualifies as a reportable sentinel event under the JCAHO's policy, the call for a root-cause analysis was automatic. The investigation involved staff from the PICU pharmacy, medical staff, and nursing staff. As this book was going to press, they'd just submitted an initial report. "[The team] found the proximate cause right away," said the risk manager. "The medication wasn't mixed properly."

The root-cause analysis team made that determination after a thorough review of the infant's medical record eliminated most other potential proximate causes. The physician's order, for instance, called for the right dose. That order was transcribed and forwarded to pharmacy correctly. The medication administration record indicated that the nurse had administered the drug as ordered. The pharmacy's unit-dose container was even labeled with the proper dose. However, lab tests on the syringe that was used to inject the child showed that the gentamicin residue inside was four times more concentrated than it should have been.

The root-cause analysis team's report outlined plans to give pharmacy staff additional training on mixing and compounding drugs. While acknowledging that the team could probably dig further into pharmacy procedures, the risk manager wasn't optimistic that much would turn up. "We have found that errors in the pharmacy happen less than one-tenth of 1 percent of the time," the risk manager noted. "This may be the best we can do."

Nonetheless, the risk-management advisory board sent the report back to the team for further analysis. "The root-cause analysis...didn't tell us if they'd done an audiogram on the child," the risk manager said, "which means they probably didn't do a [very thorough investigation.]" The report also included a note from the nursing staff denying involvement in the overdose and pointing a finger at the pharmacy. "This tells me that this nurse has no idea what we're trying to do with regard to root-cause analysis," the risk manager said. "This process is not about finger pointing. If evidence points to the pharmacy as the primary source of error, the nursing and medical staffs should help the pharmacy identify root causes, and they should look at their own procedures to determine what, if anything, kept them from preventing this overdose."

SUGGESTED READING

Books

Joint Commission on Accreditation of Healthcare Organizations. *Sentinel Events: Evaluating Cause and Planning Improvement* (Oakbrook Terrace, IL: JCAHO, 1998).

Spath, Patrice L. *Investigating Sentinel Events: How to Find and Resolve Root Causes* (Forest Grove, OR: Brown-Spath & Associates, 1998).

Wilson, PF, LD Dell, and GF Anderson, *Root Cause Analysis: A Tool for Total Quality Management* (Milwaukee: ASQC Quality Press, 1993).

Articles

Blumenthal, D. "Making medical errors into medical treasures." *JAMA* 272 (23): 1851-7 (1994).

Cohen, MR, J Senders, and NM Davis. "Failure mode and effects analysis: a novel approach to avoiding dangerous medication errors and accidents." *Hosp Pharm* 29: 205-11 (1994).

Cooper, JB, RS Newbower, and RJ Ritz. "An Analysis of major errors and equipment failures in anesthesia management: Considerations for prevention and detection." *Anesthesiology* 60 (1): 34-42 (1995).

Dew, JR. "In search of the root cause." *Qual Prog* 24 (3): 97-102.

Spath, Patrice L. "How to Conduct a Thorough Sentinel Event Investigation." *Journal of Healthcare Risk Management.* Fall 1998: 5–6.

Struck, Karen. "When has the Cause Analysis Reached the Root?" *Journal of Healthcare Risk Management.* Fall 1998: 6–10.

Useful Forms

The next few pages contain forms that may help your organization track adverse events and follow-up on the improvement initiatives generated by the root-cause analysis process. Healthcare organizations and professionals may reprint these forms for internal use. Reprinting for all other uses requires permission. Reprinting these forms for sale or for use in any other for-profit ventures is prohibited.

Adverse/sentinel event report

Categories of incidents (circle as appropriate)	Unexpected adverse outcomes (circle as appropriate)
patient fall procedure variance burn or other patient injury operating-room event operating-room variance material/equipment-related incident medication variance unexpected complication of outpatient care patient, staff member, or visitor attacked/raped infant abducted or discharged to wrong family procedure performed on wrong patient procedure performed on wrong body part transfusion with contaminated blood product patient suicide other: _____ (describe) near miss, any of above: _____ (describe)	hemolytic transfusion reaction transfusion-related infection motor weakness brain damage sensory nerve injury unplanned loss or impairment of reproductive organ loss or impairment of sensory organ unexpected death unexpected re-operation unexpected loss of limb, total or partial loss of limb use birth injury other: _____ (describe) near miss, any of above: _____ (describe)

Describe the event (state significant facts in chronological order)

Event date: Event time:

What caused this event?

_____

Name: Phone:

Department: Date submitted to department head/CI rep:

A department head or continuous-improvement representative should complete the rest of this form and forward it to the risk management department.

Adverse/sentinel event report (continued)

Comments of department head or continuous-improvement representative:

Is root-cause analysis necessary or required? ❑ Yes ❑ No ❑ Unknown
(If yes, or if risk management orders root-cause analysis, report findings and improvement plans within 30 days. See the back of this form for more information.)

Systems related? ❑ Yes ❑ No

Peer-review category* I II III IV (circle one)

Practitioner related?* ❑ Yes ❑ No

Sentinel event?* ❑ Yes ❑ No

Patient complaint? ❑ Yes ❑ No

Injury classification* none/minor temporary
long-term/permanent unknown (circle one)

Disability classification* none/minor temporary
long-term/permanent unknown (circle one)

*See definitions and guidelines section for explanation

Name: Phone:

Department: Date submitted to risk management:

Inpatient record number: **Outpatient record number:**

This is a confidential document. DO NOT release information contained in this document to unauthorized individuals. This information may be used to assist attorneys representing this organization's interests during litigation. Store copies of this document in departmental CI files only. DO NOT file by patient name, social security number, or any other patient identifier. DO NOT place this report in the patient's record.

Adverse/sentinel event report (continued)

Definitions and guidelines applicable to this reporting form:

Sentinel event: An occurrence that requires intensive assessment including a root-cause analysis. A sentinel event includes but may not be limited to "an unexpected occurrence or variation involving serious physical or psychological injury, or the risk thereof" (JCAHO definition).

Adverse event: An event or outcome in which a patient suffers a lack of improvement, injury, or illness that is unexpected or more severe than that ordinarily experienced by patients with a similar condition or undergoing similar procedures.

Peer-review categories:

Non-practitioner related: These events derive from factors that are intrinsic to the patient (e.g., underlying disease, biologic/anatomic variation, hypersensitivity reaction in the absence of allergic history, etc.), to institutional support functions (e.g., delay in processing of lab tests, x-rays, chart requests, etc.), or to care provided outside this organization. Data in this category will not reveal opportunities to improve practitioner performance, but may reveal trends that are useful for departmental or organizational management.

Practitioner-related: The four categories listed below include events that, individually or in aggregate, are related to specific healthcare practitioners. Data derived from these categories will help identify opportunities to enhance the quality, effectiveness, and/or efficiency of care.

Category I: Predictable event within the standard of care. "Predictable" means that the event was anticipated and is well known, widely reported in the literature, and relatively common. "Within the standard of care" means that care was provided in accordance with contemporary standards of the specialty and the department.

Category II: Unpredictable event within the standard of care. "Unpredictable" means that the event is uncommon and was unanticipated, but has been described in the literature (or by medical staff) as occurring in cases where standards of care are met. (NOTE: Events in Category II are not more serious than events in Category I; both indicate instances in which treatment met accepted standards of care.)

Category III: Marginal deviation from the standard of care. This category indicates that the quality of care fell slightly below contemporary standards of the specialty or the department.

Category IV: Significant deviation from the standard of care. Events in this category represent gross deviations from contemporary standards of the specialty or the department.

Adverse/sentinel event report (continued)

Classification of injury or disability:

None or minor: Event does not slow or affect patient's recovery, health, and/or general well-being. Examples might include surgery for perforated appendix with no resulting delay in recovery, missed diagnosis of a fracture that is recognized later with no resulting deformity, delayed recovery from anesthesia not impeding overall recovery.

Temporary: Event has minimal effect on patient's recovery, health, and/or general well-being. Examples might include fall with laceration or fracture, appendectomy with a single postoperative episode of sepsis, delayed union of fracture, and incisional hernia.

Long-term/permanent: Event significantly effects a patient's recovery, health, and/or general well-being. Examples might include fall resulting in neurological injury, forearm fracture with loss of motion in wrist or elbow, inadvertent post-operative retention of a foreign object, loss of thumb or finger, anesthesia-related cardiac or respiratory arrest, loss of life from something other than terminal illness or injury.

Guidelines for protecting confidentiality of incident reports:

1. Treat this report as a confidential document.
2. Segregate sentinel/adverse event reports from general files and limit access to them.
3. DO NOT file by patient name, social security number, or other patient identifier.
4. Strictly limit report copying and distribution.
5. DO NOT place a copy of this report in the patient's record.
6. DO NOT state in the patient's record that an incident report was completed.
7. Limit the content of the report to facts. Do not draw conclusions or assign blame.

Report results of root-cause analysis and planned improvements (attach additional pages as needed):

Root-cause analysis action plan & improvement-tracking form

RCA identifier #: _____ Event description: _____

Root causes and improvement plan (attach RCA report and supporting documents)	Improvement coordinator or CI/QI representative	How will you monitor and measure effective-ness of improvements?	Additional comments	Follow-up due on...	Expected date of completion
Root cause(s): Planned improvement(s):	Name: Phone: Email:				
Root cause(s): Planned improvement(s):	Name: Phone: Email:				
Root cause(s): Planned improvement(s):	Name: Phone: Email:				
Root cause(s): Planned improvement(s):	Name: Phone: Email:				

After finishing a root-cause analysis, please complete this form and submit it to the risk management department, along with your root-cause analysis report. This form will help the risk management department, and others, track the progress of improvement initiatives, which are vital to quality of care. The information in this document is confidential.

Designing and Implementing Improvement Proposals

Addressing root causes

In the context of adverse clinical outcomes—like medication errors and other adverse drug events—root causes represent nothing less than flaws in the way that an organization cares for patients. Once organizations identify the root causes of adverse events, therefore, they must take concrete, measurable steps to address them and stop patterns of error from repeating themselves. The Joint Commission on Accreditation of Healthcare Organizations (JCAHO) recognizes this fact, which is why its sentinel event policy insists that root-cause analyses include an action plan for improvement.

Operational changes should not be treated lightly, though—particularly when they affect quality of care. It's important to monitor the results of improvement initiatives—to confirm that they're having the effects intended, and to ensure that they are not having an unexpected impact elsewhere along the continuum of care. For example, organizations that seek to improve medication safety by having pharmacists spend more time in patient-care areas, need to ensure that quality and efficiency in the pharmacy don't suffer as a result. Organizations need to plan and test improvement initiatives carefully—identifying the likely effects on all organizational functions, then monitoring the actual impact on those functions. Whenever possible, organizations may want to stage small-scale trials, testing changes in one or two departments before enacting them across an entire facility or network.

This chapter introduces an approach to designing, testing, and implementing improvement initiatives: the FOCUS PDCA method. It also addresses challenges involved in collecting performance data and looks at innovative collection methods. It introduces tools that, along with those discussed in Chapter 3, can help healthcare facilities collect, organize, analyze, and display performance data effectively. And it concludes with a case study that describes how a Florida hospital used event-monitoring software and traditional quality-improvement techniques to address a series of adverse drug events (ADE).

FOCUS PDCA: An emphasis on proactive analysis

The FOCUS PDCA approach to quality improvement builds upon one of the earliest systematic techniques for controlling quality: the PDCA method (see Figure 4.1). Walter Shewart, an early quality pioneer, developed the PDCA method in the 1920s. In the 1950s, W. Edwards Deming popularized the approach among Japanese manufacturers— which is why it is sometimes called "The Deming Cycle."

Organizations can apply Shewart's and Deming's four-stage PDCA process proactively, but most view it as a reactive tool. Rather than using the process to assess and improve systems before a problem arises, they generally wait for signs of an adverse event or outcome and apply the PDCA method in response.

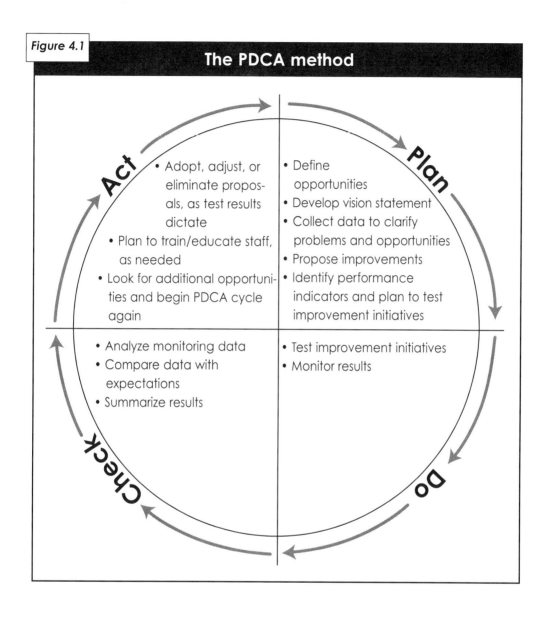

Figure 4.1

The PDCA method

Act
- Adopt, adjust, or eliminate proposals, as test results dictate
- Plan to train/educate staff, as needed
- Look for additional opportunities and begin PDCA cycle again

Plan
- Define opportunities
- Develop vision statement
- Collect data to clarify problems and opportunities
- Propose improvements
- Identify performance indicators and plan to test improvement initiatives

Check
- Analyze monitoring data
- Compare data with expectations
- Summarize results

Do
- Test improvement initiatives
- Monitor results

FOCUS PDCA makes the proactive potential of the basic Shewart/Deming approach more explicit. In the process, it turns an effective quality-assurance tool into a powerful vehicle for continuous quality improvement (see Chapter 3, Exhibit E, for more on distinctions between the two). FOCUS PDCA challenges organizations to seek out improvement opportunities (see Figure 4.2) and promote change—even

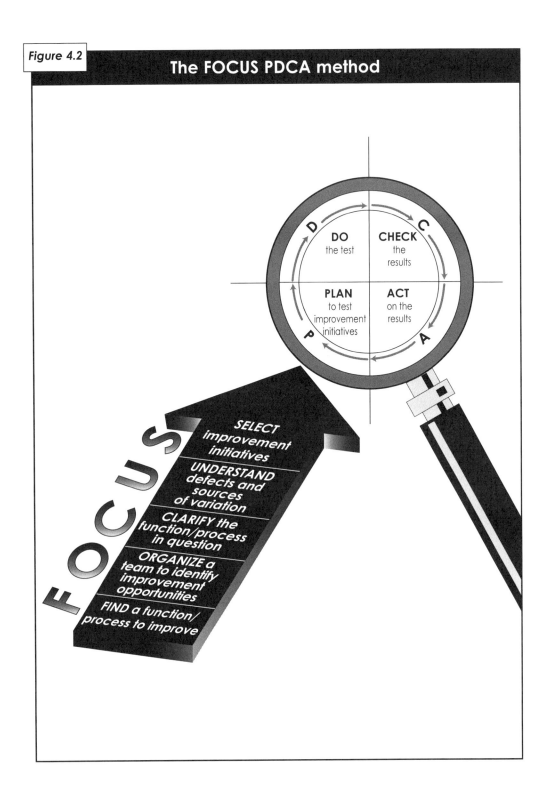

Figure 4.2

The FOCUS PDCA method

in systems and processes that appear to be running smoothly. It is founded upon the assumption that a system can always run better.

FOCUS PDCA in the context of root-cause analysis

Though it is largely reactive in nature, the root-cause analysis process mirrors the FOCUS phase of FOCUS PDCA. By the time root-cause analysis teams have completed the investigative process that's outlined in Chapter 3, they are generally ready to implement improvement initiatives—which is the primary focus of the PDCA phase. The following summary of the FOCUS phase, therefore, reviews some information on reactive root-cause analysis from the last chapter, but it also recasts that information in a context that emphasizes the potential for proactive systems analysis to prevent the events that create a need for root-cause analysis.

FOCUS: Find a process to improve

Ideally, healthcare organizations seek to establish mechanisms that reveal systemic defects or minor performance variations before a patient gets hurt—mechanisms like performance measures, monitoring systems, and an organizational culture that seeks out opportunities to change and improve. But when an adverse drug event (ADE) or some other serious incident does occur, an organization's first challenge is to define the processes that played a causal role.

In the case of medication errors and other ADE, several factors tend to play a role: equipment and materials, policies and procedures, work environment, education and training, communication, and access to information. The organization must determine which factors, processes, and functions were, or could have been, involved and make changes that are designed to prevent similar occurrences in the future.

Applied proactively, systems analysis becomes more speculative. Organizations must identify components of a process or function that seem likely to cause performance variation and launch improvement initiatives that are designed to prevent adverse events from occurring.

FOCUS: Organize a team

Analysis teams that are responsible either for reactive investigation of an ADE or for proactive identification of opportunities to improve medication safety must have firsthand knowledge of the process(es) that they are evaluating. In both cases, this means securing the participation of doctors, nurses, and pharmacists in an inquiry—as well as a risk or quality manager who is familiar with statistical analysis and can facilitate the investigative process. It's also important for teams to have decision-making authority, which means that support from the organization's senior management is crucial.

FOCUS: Clarify the process in question

Once an organization has identified key processes and organized a team to improve them, that team must carefully chart each step in the process(es) under examination. Recruiting team members who have a relevant mix of skills and expertise is an important first step. Flow charts can often supplement their knowledge and assist the clarification process—as can interviews with, and surveys of, others involved in the function(s) in question (see Chapter 3 for more on these tools).

FOCUS: Understand sources of variation

Clarifying each step in the process under investigation often helps the team begin to identify gaps, inefficiencies, defects, and risk areas—aspects of that process that seem likely to prompt performance variations. As they identify such flaws, it's important for team members to ask themselves what, if anything, caused them. They must peel away as many causal layers as possible to uncover the fundamental root causes of performance variation within that process, function, or system. Cause-and-effect diagrams and flow charts are among the tools that can help their analysis (see Chapter 3).

FOCUS: Select improvement initiatives

Once teams understand the root causes of performance variation, they can begin to propose and design improvement initiatives. If teams develop a number of improvement proposals, or if they locate more systemic defects than they can realistically address, pareto charts and decision matrices can help them determine which problems are most pressing and/or which change proposals are likely to have the most significant effect (see Chapter 3).

PDCA: Data-driven change, measurable improvement

Healthcare organizations often approach change cautiously—and they should. Not all change leads to improvement, as the Coca Cola Company learned after it introduced New Coke. But, unlike miscalculations in the business sector, mistakes in healthcare can place patients' lives in jeopardy. That's why it's crucial for healthcare organizations to track performance indicators that can help them make educated decisions about the need for change. And, that's why they must have the means to monitor the results of improvement initiatives. If an initiative is not having the expected effect, or if it is having an unexpected impact on other functions, organizations need to react quickly—before the quality of patient care is affected significantly. The FOCUS phase of FOCUS PDCA provides a systematic, data-driven method for identifying improvement needs and designing change initiatives; it is the analysis phase of the process. The PDCA phase, described below, offers a proven method for implementing, evaluating, and, as necessary, adjusting initiatives to make them as effective as possible.

PDCA: Plan to test/implement initiatives

A change is not necessarily an improvement, and, because changes can affect quality of care, organizations often hold small-scale trials of a new process before implementing it widely. Sometimes called pilots, these test runs allow the organization to control or minimize the impact of a new method or procedure until there's clear evidence that the effects will be positive. Also, because they are limited in scope, trial runs are often a more cost-effective way to experiment with new policies and procedures than immediate, full-scale implementation.

Regardless of whether improvement teams choose to stage a trial, it is crucial that its members develop an action plan to guide their implementation and evaluation efforts (see Figure 4.3). Effective action plans include seven basic components:

1. A mission statement that defines a specific, measurable objective;
2. An overview of tactics (change initiatives) that will help the team fulfill its objective;
3. Clear, measurable expectations regarding targeted results;
4. Identification of performance indicators to measure actual results against expectations;

Figure 4.3

Sample QI action plan

QI Action Plan

QI Facilitator: Launch Date:

Mission Statement:

Improvement Tactics	Performance Indicators	Data Sources & Collection Methods	Analysis Due	Results & Recommendations
tactic: coordinator: targeted result:			prelim: final:	
tactic: coordinator: targeted result:			prelim: final:	
tactic: coordinator: targeted result:			prelim: final:	
tactic: coordinator: targeted result:			prelim: final:	

5. An explanation of data-collection mechanisms to be used in monitoring those indicators;
6. Designations of responsibility for each action item or tactic in the plan; and
7. A timeline for staging preliminary and final assessments of each change initiative.

The planning process should include careful consideration of all possible direct and indirect effects of a change initiative. Patient-care functions and processes are often interconnected, but not always in obvious ways. Adjustments to one may produce effects in others, and, if team members don't commit time and resources to anticipating, addressing, and monitoring those effects, a negative impact in one area can negate important gains in another.

PDCA: Do the test/implement change

Once the team has outlined its tactics, assigned responsibilities, and settled on a timeline for each initiative, it is ready to implement the proposed changes. Depending on the size of the team and the number of initiatives in progress, team members may want to separate themselves into smaller work groups for this phase. If so, periodic meetings of the full team will help keep the overall project on track, will allow work group members to seek input, and will provide a forum for reporting and discussing preliminary findings.

PDCA: Check the results

When the trial run (or the initial phase of a full-scale implementation), is complete, the team should analyze the performance monitoring data that it collected and compare its findings against its improvement goals. A wide range of statistical-analysis tools (see pages 80–92 and 123–145) are available to assist this process.

PDCA: Act on the results

If the results of an improvement plan are unsatisfactory, the team may need to reconsider or refine proposed changes and repeat the PDCA cycle. If, however, change initiatives meet or exceed expectations, team members should take steps to enact them across the organization. Enactment may involve working with hospital leadership to revise existing policies and procedures, developing staff-retraining initiatives, and other activities.

Effective benchmarking and data collection

Accurate, reliable data collection and event reporting are crucial to the success of improvement initiatives. Unless teams have benchmarking data that gives them an accurate picture of performance, they can't develop effective improvement proposals. And if they can't get data that allows them to compare the effects of new policies and procedures against their benchmarks and expectations, it's difficult to judge the efficacy of change initiatives.

Traditionally, improvement teams have collected performance and outcomes data via chart review—a process that's labor intensive, time consuming, and, because it relies on human observation, error prone (see Chapter 1 for more on "the human factor"). Furthermore, where adverse events are concerned, improvement and root-cause analysis teams have long relied on incident data that's reported voluntarily, by people who were involved in an incident or who witnessed it. But voluntary reporting is widely acknowledged to be unreliable—particularly if the people providing information believe that they may face legal or disciplinary action for speaking up. Therefore, as efforts have progressed to encourage a systems-analysis approach to error prevention in healthcare, organizations have sought alternatives to these traditional information-gathering tools. A few promising approaches have resulted.

Monitoring event indicators

Some organizations define specific risk indicators—that is, procedures, outcomes, and other treatment patterns and trends—that suggest an adverse event occurred. Analysts and coders in the organization's HIM department monitor chart documentation for these risk indicators and notify the risk-management or quality staff when they appear. This approach eliminates a key barrier to voluntary reporting, for, unlike caregivers, coders and analysts don't risk being blamed, disciplined, or held legally responsible for the adverse events they report.

Once risk or quality managers are notified of cases that contain risk indicators, they investigate to determine: 1) whether an adverse event did occur; 2) whether the occurrence is similar to other incidents and part of a pattern of performance variation; and 3) whether improvement opportunities exist. The hospital profiled in Chapter 3 (see pages 93–102) employs this method to identify possible sentinel events (see Figure 3.7 for a list of this hospital's risk indicators).

Monitoring for event indicators still requires a significant commitment of time and resources, and it is not a foolproof process. To gather follow-up information, for instance, risk and quality managers often rely on chart reviews, interviews, and other methods that are labor intensive and sometimes unreliable. But the risk indicators make their search for adverse events more targeted and efficient than if they relied on random chart reviews and voluntary reporting by caregivers.

Tracking events and indicators electronically

A number of organizations use computer technology to expedite the monitoring and reporting process, and to improve the reliability of that process by limiting the effects of "the human factor." These systems tend to focus on tracking either actual adverse events or event indicators. Exhibits I and J provide brief descriptions of two such systems.

More tools to assist analysis

Chapter 3 introduced tools in the context of reactive root-cause analysis (see pages 80–92) that organizations can also use during more proactive improvement initiatives. In addition, improvement teams often use the tools discussed below to help them organize, analyze, and display data effectively.

Bar graphs

Bar graphs allow analysis teams to compare different sets of data or different components of one data set. They allow teams to track trends and identify patterns than can help them establish improvement priorities and target initiatives effectively. For example, if a team were investigating missed medication doses, a bar graph would allow team members to display raw data so that they could easily compare missed-dose totals per ward, per work shift, or per week.

Depending on their analysis needs, improvement teams usually employ one of three common types of bar graph: 1) simple bar graphs; 2) clustered bar graphs; and 3) stratified bar graphs.

Exhibit I

Event-monitoring software

University Community Hospital (UCH) in Tampa, Florida, relies on innovative event-tracking software (see the UCH case study, pages 146–152) to gather data on a wide range of adverse events, including medication errors and ADE. The system gathers information on adverse events from sources all over the hospital and consolidates it in a single database.

Because it tracks actual adverse events, a system like UCH's is only effective if incident reporting is reliable. Organizations that employ such systems often establish confidential reporting channels or offer immunity (or limited immunity) from punishment to staff who volunteer information about an incident. Representatives from Tampa-based Management Prescriptives, Inc. (MPI), the company that developed UCH's software, say that, as staff at their client hospitals grow comfortable with the system and with the nonpunitive objectives of the reporting process, their willingness to report events increases.

Exhibit J

Indicator-monitoring software

Brigham and Women's Hospital (BWH) in Boston and LDS Hospital in Salt Lake City use computer technology in a slightly different way than Tampa-based University Community Hospital does (See Exhibit I). BWH and LDS have developed computerized systems that track adverse-event indicators—rather than actual adverse events.[*] These systems are linked to databases where treatment information is stored, and they are programmed to flag cases that contain the tell-tale signs of an adverse event—such as:

- orders to stop use of a drug or to change drugs in mid-treatment, which may indicate that an ADR occurred;
- orders for common allergy antidotes (like an antihistamine), which could indicate an allergic reaction; or
- abnormal lab-test results, which might suggest treatment isn't progressing normally or as expected.

The principle behind these systems is the same as for systems that rely on analysts and coders to flag risk indicators. However, an employee is more likely than a computer to overlook a risk indicator, and computers can be programmed to track more indicators than an employee can reliably monitor.

---

[*] *Developed in 1989, the computerized-monitoring system at LDS Hospital has served as an industry model. For more information, see: David C. Classen, et. al., "Adverse Drug Events in Hospitalized Patients," JAMA 277 (4): 301-6 (1997).*

Simple bar graph

A simple bar graph (see Figure 4.4a) is useful for analyzing data that cannot be (or does not need to be) arranged into sub-categories. Each bar in the graph displays data from a discrete data set (e.g., one bar for missed doses in January, one for February, etc.)—making it easy to compare totals for, and identify patterns in, the data collected. The graph in Figure 4.4a, for instance, displays data on the occurrence of ADE and potential ADE at two Boston area hospitals (see Chapters 1 and 2 for more information on this research) during key stages of the medication-use process: ordering, transcribing, dispensing, and administering. It indicates that the vast majority of ADE and potential ADE occur during the ordering and administration stages—information that might help an improvement team prioritize or target possible change initiatives.

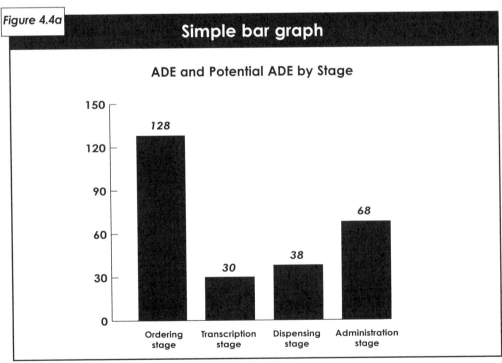

Figure 4.4a

Simple bar graph

ADE and Potential ADE by Stage

Source: "Table 6.—Stages of Primary Errors Associated With Preventable and Potential Adverse Drug Events" in David W. Bates, David J. Cullen, et al., "Incidence of Adverse Drug Events and Potential Adverse Drug Events," JAMA 274 (1): 3 (1995).

Clustered bar graph

If the total displayed in each bar of a simple bar graph can be divided into useful subtotals, a team might choose to display the data using a clustered bar graph (see Figure 4.4b). The clusters of bars in Figure 4.4b display subcategories of the data that were shown in each single bar in Figure 4.4a. (Whereas Figure 4.4a focuses on total ADE and potential ADE, Figure 4.4b separates that data into three subtotals: preventable ADE, intercepted potential ADE, and potential ADE not intercepted.) The sum of the subtotals displayed in each cluster of narrow bars in Figure 4.4b is equal to the total represented in the corresponding single bar in Figure 4.4a. Likewise, if the narrow bars in each cluster were stacked, they would reach the same height as the

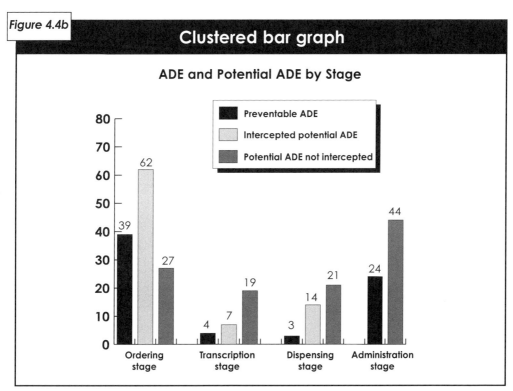

Figure 4.4b

Clustered bar graph

ADE and Potential ADE by Stage

Legend:
- Preventable ADE
- Intercepted potential ADE
- Potential ADE not intercepted

Source: "Table 6.—Stages of Primary Errors Associated With Preventable and Potential Adverse Drug Events" in David W. Bates, David J. Cullen, et al., "Incidence of Adverse Drug Events and Potential Adverse Drug Events," JAMA 274 (1): 33 (1995).

corresponding single bar in Figure 4.4a. Clustered bar graphs are useful for displaying data in a format that emphasizes the relative impact of subtotals, but still allows for some comparison of totals.

Stratified bar graph

Like a clustered bar graph, the stratified bar graph allows a team to display subtotals. But rather than using a separate bar for each subtotal, a stratified bar graph divides one bar into proportional segments (Figure 4.4c). Whereas a clustered bar graph calls attention to subtotals, a stratified bar graph emphasizes overall totals, while still allowing for some comparison of subtotals.

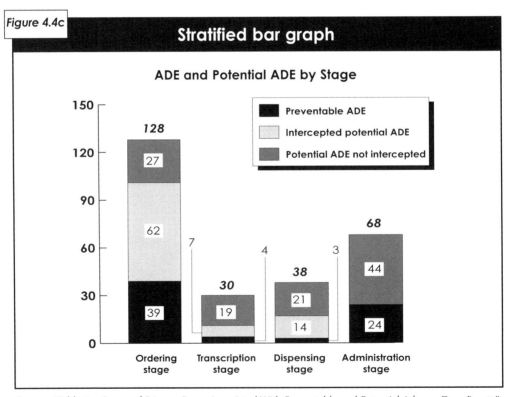

Figure 4.4c

Stratified bar graph

ADE and Potential ADE by Stage

Source: "Table 6.—Stages of Primary Errors Associated With Preventable and Potential Adverse Drug Events" in David W. Bates, David J. Cullen, et al., "Incidence of Adverse Drug Events and Potential Adverse Drug Events," JAMA 274 (1): 33 (1995).

Brainstorming

Improvement teams generally brainstorm when they want to generate as many ideas as possible on a particular subject. For instance, brainstorming might be good way to begin analyzing a system for possible defects or identifying possible improvement initiatives.

Brainstorming sessions should be spontaneous, unstructured, lively, and brief (i.e., no longer than an hour). The session facilitator should introduce the topic and the session's objectives, then open the floor to ideas. As the session progresses, the facilitator should ask questions and introduce sub-topics that will guide the group in useful directions. To encourage creativity and input, team members and the facilitator should withhold judgment on ideas until the brainstorming session is complete.

Brainstorming sessions should include people with direct knowledge of the subject under consideration. But it may also be useful to involve people with little or no relevant expertise; they're often the ones to ask questions or make off-beat suggestions that propel the group's thinking in innovative directions. Sessions should include enough people to generate a lot of ideas, without being so big that the meeting becomes unmanageable. Six to twelve people is generally an effective size.

Check sheets

A check sheet is a grid that allows improvement teams to organize and tally performance data (see Figure 4.5). Check sheets do not reveal causal information. However, they can help improvement teams compare rates and patterns of occurrence, and they may help teams set improvement priorities. Check sheets are often used to tally raw data, which can then be displayed in charts and graphs that facilitate more sophisticated systems analysis.

Figure 4.5

Check sheet

	Missed Doses (per work shift)					
	Mon.	Tues.	Wed.	Thurs.	Fri.	Totals (weekly)
Days	✓✓✓	✓✓✓✓✓	✓	✓✓	✓✓✓✓✓✓	17
Evenings	✓✓✓✓✓	✓✓✓✓✓	✓✓✓	✓✓✓✓		17
Overnights	✓✓✓✓✓✓✓	✓✓✓✓	✓✓✓✓✓✓	✓✓✓✓✓ ✓✓✓✓✓	✓✓✓✓✓	32
Totals (daily)	15	14	10	16	11	66

Hypothetical scenario. Not based on real data.

Histograms

A histogram is a form of bar graph that's useful for comparing patterns of actual occurrence against a specific standard or set of expectations. For instance, if a physician prescribes a medication that must be taken every six hours, a histogram could show how well the patient is complying with that treatment regimen (see Figures 4.6a and 4.6b).

Analysis of Figure 4.6a indicates that, during the first week of treatment the patient complied with the every-six-hours regimen—though a few doses were taken late or early. However, Figure 4.6b suggests that, in the second week of treatment, the patient was less compliant, often waiting more than six hours between doses. (Note: For histogram analysis to be helpful, an event needs to occur quite a few times. It's

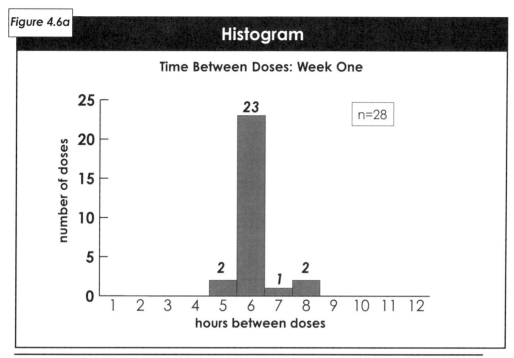

Hypothetical scenario. Not based on real data.

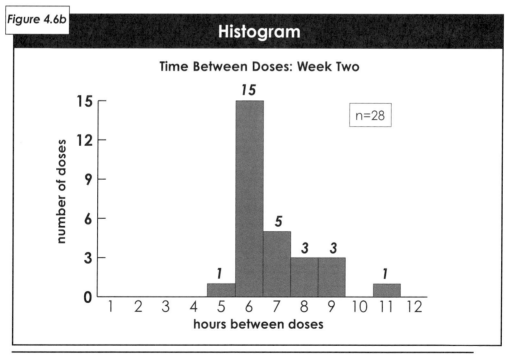

Hypothetical scenario. Not based on real data.

generally harder to identify significant patterns in data from small sample sizes.)

Histograms are useful, in part, because the pattern formed by the array of bars can, at a glance, provide important information about the process under examination. For instance:

- A cluster of bars that peaks in the middle and has a narrow base suggests there is little performance variation in the process under examination (see Figure 4.7a).

- A cluster that peaks in the middle but has a wide base indicates a lot of performance variation (see Figure 4.7b).

- Histograms that peak on the left or right are known as "skewed histograms." They indicate either that something happened to produce unexpected results or that data was left out during creation of the histogram (see Figure 4.7c).

- Combining incompatible data sets often generates a histogram with two peaks—what's known as a bimodal histogram (see Figure 4.7d). The data from these sets should be separated and redisplayed in two histograms.

The first example (Figure 4.7a), which is sometimes called a "normal histogram," indicates that a process is proceeding largely as expected. The other examples suggest a need for improvement.

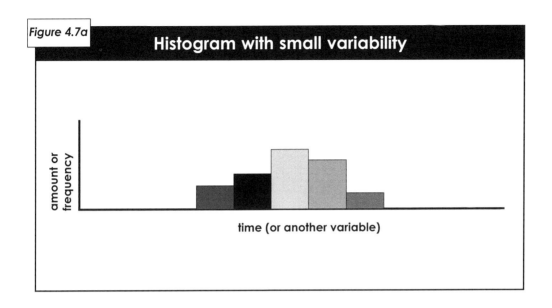

Figure 4.7a — Histogram with small variability

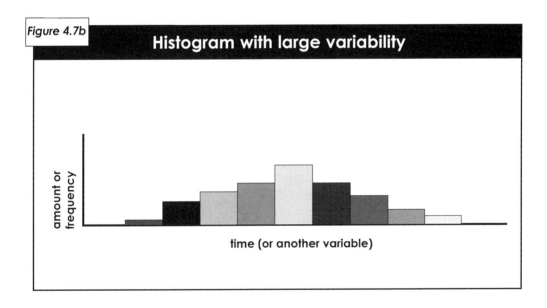

Figure 4.7b — Histogram with large variability

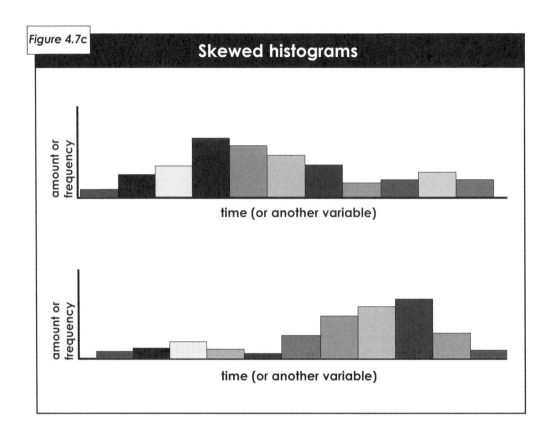

Figure 4.7c — Skewed histograms

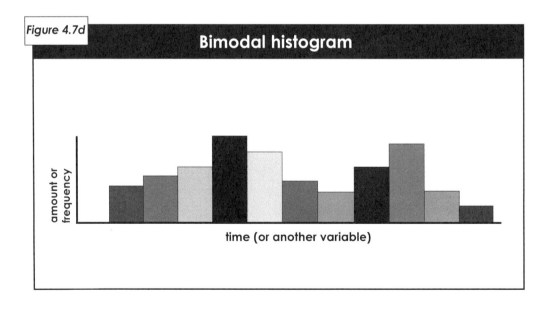

Figure 4.7d — Bimodal histogram

Pie charts

Like bar graphs, a pie chart is a comparative tool that displays relationships between data sets, or between component parts (subcategories) of one data set. These charts may help improvement teams set priorities—by revealing, for instance, where adverse events are having the greatest impact, or which aspects of a system or process are most frequently a source of performance variation (see Figure 4.8).

Analysis of the chart in Figure 4.8 indicates that poor dissemination of drug knowledge was the most common root cause of ADE and potential ADE in a study at two Boston-area hospitals (see Chapters 1 and 2 for more on this study). The study uncovered 16 root causes in all, which are arrayed clockwise and in descending order of frequency on the chart. A stratified bar graph (see page 128) could conceivably display the same information, but once the bar has to be divided more than three or four times, it can be hard to read and differences between data sets may become less obvious.

Unlike bar graphs, pie charts are not very effective for displaying patterns of occurrence over time. If, for instance, a hospital wanted to track medication errors per month in the ICU, a bar graph with 12 bars would allow the organization to study a year's worth of monthly totals. Patterns within the data might not be as obvious if the data were displayed in 12 pie-chart segments. Pie charts are effective for displaying before-and-after data, though—especially if the chart format highlights the segments that depict significant or relevant changes (see Figure 4.9).

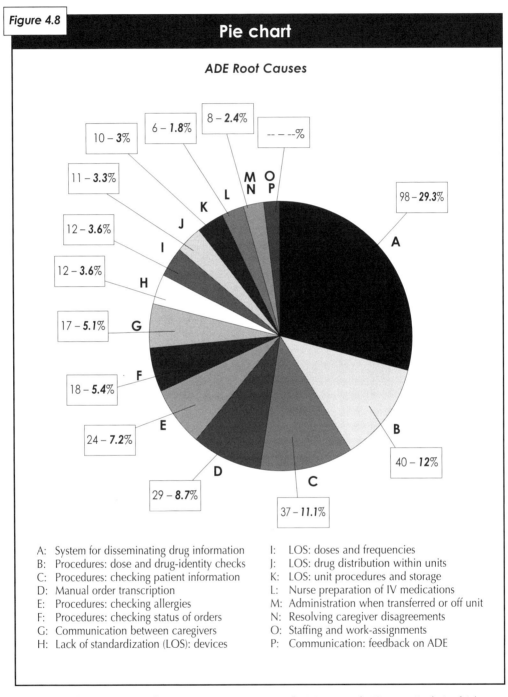

Figure 4.8

Pie chart

ADE Root Causes

8 – **2.4%**

6 – **1.8%**

10 – **3%**

-- – --%

11 – **3.3%**

98 – **29.3%**

12 – **3.6%**

12 – **3.6%**

17 – **5.1%**

18 – **5.4%**

24 – **7.2%**

40 – **12%**

29 – **8.7%**

37 – **11.1%**

A: System for disseminating drug information
B: Procedures: dose and drug-identity checks
C: Procedures: checking patient information
D: Manual order transcription
E: Procedures: checking allergies
F: Procedures: checking status of orders
G: Communication between caregivers
H: Lack of standardization (LOS): devices

I: LOS: doses and frequencies
J: LOS: drug distribution within units
K: LOS: unit procedures and storage
L: Nurse preparation of IV medications
M: Administration when transferred or off unit
N: Resolving caregiver disagreements
O: Staffing and work-assignments
P: Communication: feedback on ADE

Source: "Table 7.—Systems Failures," in Lucian L. Leape, David W. Bates, et al., "Systems Analysis of Adverse Drug Events," JAMA 274 (1): 41 (1995).

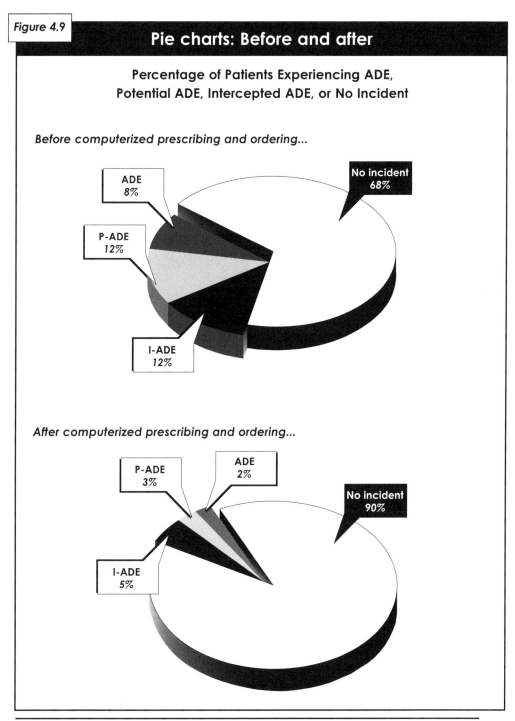

Figure 4.9

Pie charts: Before and after

Percentage of Patients Experiencing ADE, Potential ADE, Intercepted ADE, or No Incident

Before computerized prescribing and ordering...

No incident
68%

ADE
8%

P-ADE
12%

I-ADE
12%

After computerized prescribing and ordering...

P-ADE
3%

ADE
2%

No incident
90%

I-ADE
5%

Hypothetical scenario. Not based on actual data.

Radar charts

A radar chart displays before-and-after data, measuring variables at different points, showing how those measurements change over time, and allowing for comparison between variables. For instance, this tool might be especially useful for displaying changes in attitudes as reflected by survey data (see Figure 4.10).

The radar chart in Figure 4.10 gauges the theoretical effect on patient attitudes of a highly publicized medication error. It indicates that patients saw improvement over time in all assessment areas except those associated with quality of care. Before the medication error, for instance, quality of non-emergency care (Assessment Area B) scored 4.2 on a scale of 5. After the error that score dropped to 3.1. By comparing this dip in patient confidence with data related to the other hospital functions, hospital administrators can begin to identify improvement and public-relations priorities.

Run charts

A run chart is a form of line graph that, like some bar graphs, displays patterns in data over time (see Figure 4.11). It is useful for revealing outcome trends and may help improvement teams begin to generate hypotheses about why a particular performance variation occurs. The run chart in Figure 4.11, for instance, looks at a hypothetical correlation between medication errors and shift length at a hospital where residents work 24-hour shifts. It indicates that errors occur with greater frequency toward the end of long shifts, which might prompt an improvement or root-cause analysis team to consider whether fatigue played a role in the performance variations.

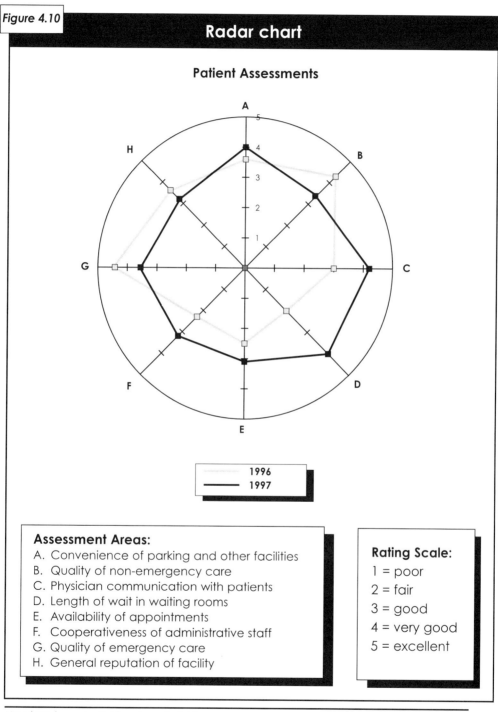

Figure 4.10

Radar chart

Patient Assessments

Assessment Areas:
A. Convenience of parking and other facilities
B. Quality of non-emergency care
C. Physician communication with patients
D. Length of wait in waiting rooms
E. Availability of appointments
F. Cooperativeness of administrative staff
G. Quality of emergency care
H. General reputation of facility

Rating Scale:
1 = poor
2 = fair
3 = good
4 = very good
5 = excellent

Hypothetical scenario. Not based on actual data.

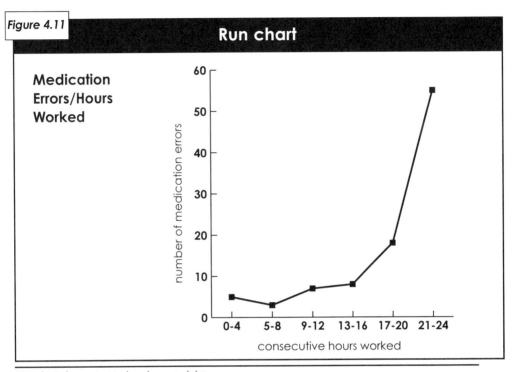

Figure 4.11

Run chart

Medication Errors/Hours Worked

number of medication errors

60
50
40
30
20
10
0

0-4 5-8 9-12 13-16 17-20 21-24

consecutive hours worked

Hypothetical scenario. Not based on actual data.

Run charts are also effective for comparing performance during a specific period of time against a long-term average or performance standard. Figure 4.12, for instance, compares monthly medication-error totals in an organization against the previous year's monthly average. Since the monthly totals only exceed the previous year's average (indicated by the dotted line) twice, this chart suggests that medication errors are occurring less frequently than before. Displaying before-and-after data in this format can be a compelling way to report the results of successful improvement initiatives.

Scatter diagrams

Scatter diagrams reveal whether a relationship exists between two variables. For instance, an organization might use a scatter diagram to

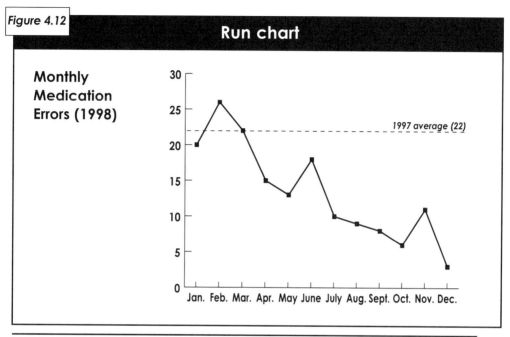

Figure 4.12

Run chart

Monthly Medication Errors (1998)

1997 average (22)

Jan. Feb. Mar. Apr. May June July Aug. Sept. Oct. Nov. Dec.

Hypothetical scenario. Not based on actual data.

determine whether there's a correlation between nurse-involvement in ADE and work experience (see Figures 4.13a–4.13e). The y-axis in each figure tracks ADE-involvement, while the x-axis indicates total years of service. The pattern created by the array of data points reveals the relationship, if any exists, between the variables.

Negative correlation

When the data points extend in relatively tight band from the upper left quadrant to the lower right quadrant of a scatter diagram, that suggests a negative correlation. In other words, Figure 4.13a suggests that nurses with more experience are less likely to be involved in an ADE. A team reviewing this diagram, therefore, might explore opportunities for improving training, supervision, and support for less-experienced nurses.

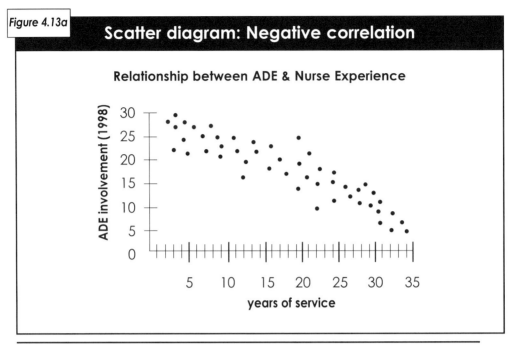

Figure 4.13a

Scatter diagram: Negative correlation

Relationship between ADE & Nurse Experience

Hypothetical scenario. Not based on actual data.

Positive correlation

When the data points extend in a relatively tight band from the lower left quadrant to the upper right quadrant of a scatter diagram, that suggests a positive correlation between variables. Figure 4.13b, for example, indicates that, as nurse experience increases, so does involvement in ADE. Common sense suggests that this is an illogical finding, and improvement teams faced with such a finding might attempt to determine whether other factors are at work. However, the findings might also suggest that older nurses aren't familiar with current safety-improvement techniques or tend to disregard accepted safety procedures—which might prompt an improvement team to propose retraining initiatives for experienced nurses.

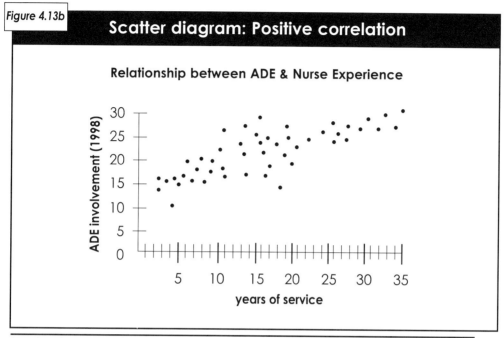

Figure 4.13b

Scatter diagram: Positive correlation

Relationship between ADE & Nurse Experience

Hypothetical scenario. Not based on actual data.

Correlation shift

If the data-point pattern forms a peak or trough in the middle of a scatter diagram, that suggests a correlation shift. Figure 4.13c, for instance, suggests that nurse involvement in ADE increases along with experience for ten years (a positive correlation), but, after ten years, the correlation becomes negative (involvement in ADE begins to decline as experience increases beyond ten years). Figure 4.13d, on the other hand, indicates the opposite scenario: an initially negative correlation that becomes positive after several years. Based on findings like these, a team might choose to target nurses for medication-safety training, supervision, and/or support at key points in their careers.

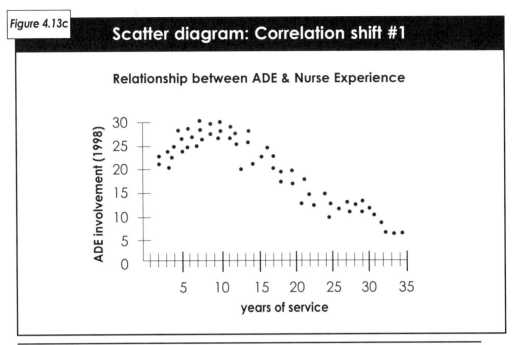

Hypothetical scenario. Not based on actual data.

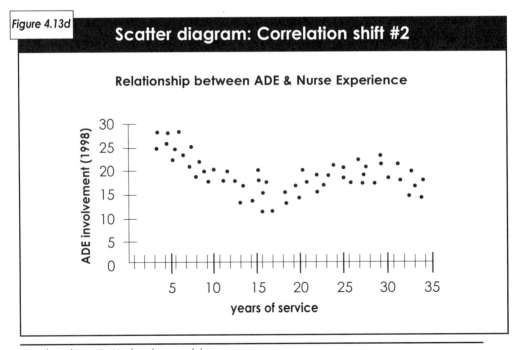

Hypothetical scenario. Not based on actual data.

No correlation

If the data points form no discernible pattern, there's no correlation between the variables. Figure 4.13e suggests, for instance, that involvement in ADE and years on the job are not related.

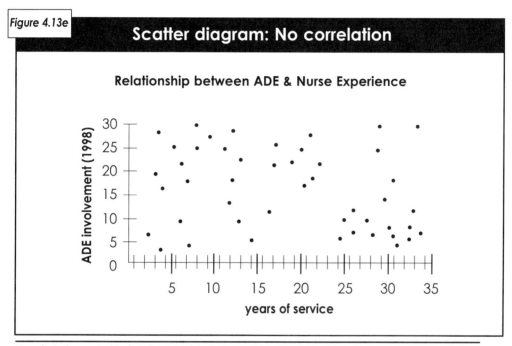

Figure 4.13e

Scatter diagram: No correlation

Relationship between ADE & Nurse Experience

Hypothetical scenario. Not based on actual data.

No substitute for experience

The principles behind systems analysis (reactive root-cause analysis and proactive quality improvement) are straightforward: 1) identify a problem or potential problem and 2) peel away causal layers to reveal the flaws in a system, process, policy, or procedure that are to blame. But just because the principles are straightforward, that does not mean the process is simple. Healthcare organizations and the modern treatments they provide rely on a complex web of interconnected functions and procedures. As with any complex system, there are a lot of ways for things to go wrong, and it's often difficult to spot inherent defects and risk points. Tracing backwards from adverse event or potential adverse event to root cause may seem as confusing as stumbling through a maze, but it can become less confounding. Whereas each new maze may be as mysterious as the last one, systems analysis becomes less daunting as organizations and individuals gain experience with the steps and the thought processes involved—and when they share the lessons that they've learned.

C A S E   S T U D Y

Hospital reduces risks and costs of drug toxicity

When it comes to data-driven quality improvement and root-cause analysis, Donna Scott is a believer. Scott is the director of quality management at University Community Hospital (UCH), which has about 550 beds across two campuses in Tampa, Florida, and admits about 19,700 patients each year. She recently advised an improvement team that investigated a series of toxic reactions to digoxin, a heart medication. The effected population was small: just 13 patients from April to June 1997, but financial data showed that treatment costs for those patients were more than $57 thousand higher than for patients with the same diagnosis but no digoxin toxicity. Traditional quality-improvement techniques and new event-monitoring software helped the hospital identify the problem and make targeted changes to its medication-use procedures. Cases of digoxin toxicity and their related costs nearly disappeared as a result.

A mystery on their hands

This string of ADE was particularly troubling, said Scott, because the reactions seemed to be happening for no good reason. In each case, the hospital's records indicated that a physician ordered an appropriate dose. Records also showed that the pharmacy dispensed the digoxin correctly, and a nurse administered each dose as ordered. But the patients still had adverse reactions, and tests showed that all had a toxic amount of digoxin in their blood. UCH assembled a team to find an explanation and propose solutions.

Getting FOCUSed: Find a function/process to improve

Though the improvement team wound up reacting to a series of actual adverse events (as opposed to identifying and addressing latent problems and defects), the investigation did not begin reactively. UCH went in search of improvement opportunities—in part to test new event-monitoring software.

The software was designed by Tampa-based Management Prescriptives, Inc.; it monitors 17 potential sources of adverse events, including use of medication. It allows MPI client hospitals to create internal databases for adverse events, but each client also has access to a central MPI database that includes adverse-event data gathered by all software users. As of late-1998, MPI had outcomes and costs data linked to about 160,000 adverse events, which its client hospitals can draw on for benchmarking and improvement initiatives.

When UCH set out to test the MPI software, the organization specifically targeted medication use. When the software turned up evidence of costly, unexplained ADE in a manageable number of cardiac patients, UCH decided to make those cases the focus of its initial investigation.

"We knew we wanted to focus on ADE," said Scott, "so we used the software to drill down and explore events: what types happened, the days of the week they happened on, where they happened, the kinds of drugs involved. Because the system ties into the costs associated with incidents, we decided to look also for something that was costing us a lot."

Getting FOCUSed: Organize a team

UCH organized a seven-person improvement team to investigate the ADE in cardiac patients. A pharmacist led the team, while Scott served as an advisor. Other team members came from the nursing staff, the quality-management department, the risk-management department, and the education department.

A representative from the medical staff did not serve on the improvement team. However, team members eventually worked with UCH's Pharmacy & Therapeutics Committee, which includes members of the medical staff, to enact improvement proposals. Despite the ultimate success of the initiative, Scott said that direct physician involvement would have been helpful and that physicians would be asked to serve on future improvement teams.

Getting FOCUSed: Clarify the function/process in question

As the investigation began, it was not clear that digoxin caused the adverse events, so the team's first challenge was to speculate about possible causes. Team members reviewed the data generated by the tracking-software and held a brainstorming session to generate ideas.

They had little to go on. Digoxin was a common thread linking each of the patients, but there was no evidence that the drug had been administered inappropriately to any patient.

Needing more answers and feeling that they'd gotten all the information they could from the software data, the team searched each patient's chart for evidence further linking the ADE. They found blood-test data indicating that all the patients had slightly elevated levels of creatinine and blood urea nitrogen (BUN)—a sign that their kidneys weren't functioning properly.

Kidneys act as a filter for the blood, removing potentially toxic substances, including some drugs, before they reach dangerous concentrations. If a patient's kidneys aren't working effectively, drugs are not removed from the body at a normal rate, and doses that would normally be safe can prove toxic. The lab-test information convinced members of the UCH improvement team that they were dealing with cases of digoxin toxicity due to reduced kidney function.

Getting FOCUSed: Understand defects and variations

Blood tests that are performed routinely on most patients admitted to UCH showed that renal function in the digoxin patients was mildly impaired—though the patients were not yet exhibiting symptoms of kidney failure. According to Scott, UCH pharmacists had access to that kidney-function data, but the hospital did not have procedures in place to facilitate pharmacist-physician consultations on that data. Team members concluded that this was a key root cause of the digoxin reactions.

Getting FOCUSed: Select improvement initiatives

The team worked with the medical and pharmacy staffs to develop procedures to guide and encourage effective interaction between pharmacists and physicians, and to help ensure that consideration of kidney function plays an appropriate role in dosing decisions. Since a blood test that measures kidney function is performed automatically on most patients at admission (the exception being a patient whose age, diagnosis, and general health make renal impairment highly unlikely), the new procedures did not require additional testing or increase hospital costs. Nor did the new procedures complicate the order-review process in the pharmacy, since pharmacists had always had access to the lab-test results.

PDCA: Assessing the new procedures

Having the event-monitoring software in place simplified the PDCA phase of UCH's improvement initiative. Once the pharmacy and medical staffs began using the new procedures, the improvement team monitored the data on medication-use outcomes and ADE-related costs that the software is designed to collect. Scott says team members saw positive trends almost immediately (see Figures 4.14a–4.14c). The number of toxic reactions to digoxin declined sharply, as did the costs associated with such ADE. Toxic reactions to other medications processed by the kidneys also dropped significantly—from nearly 80 occurrences in April 1997 to fewer than 20 incidents per month in early 1998.

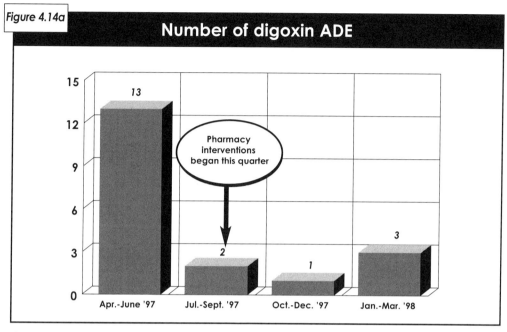

Source: University Community Hospital

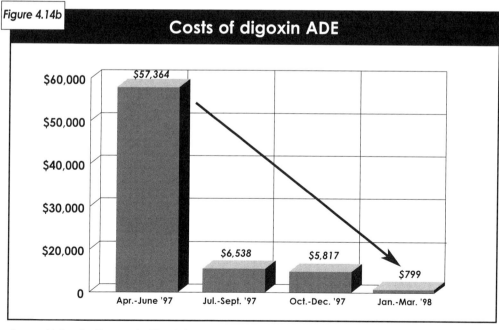

Source: University Community Hospital

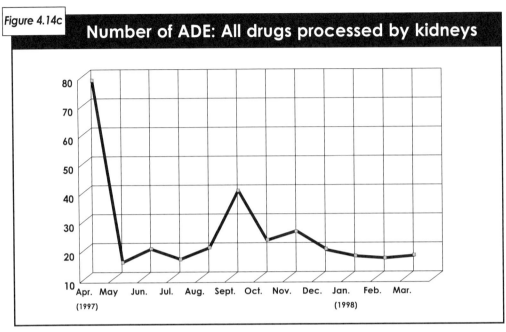

Figure 4.14c

Number of ADE: All drugs processed by kidneys

Source: University Community Hospital

S U G G E S T E D   R E A D I N G

Books:

Leape, Lucian L., Andrea Kabcenell, Donald M. Berwick, and Jane Roessner. *Reducing Adverse Drug Events* (Boston: Institute for Healthcare Improvement, 1998).

Joint Commission on Accreditation of Healthcare Organizations. *Framework for Improving Performance: From Principles to Practice* (Oakbrook Terrace, IL: JCAHO, 1997).

Articles:

Berwick, Donald M. "Continuous improvement as an ideal in health care." *N Engl J Med.* 320: 53-6 (1989).

Bradbury, K. "Prevention of medication errors: Developing a continuous–quality-improvement approach." *Mt Sinai J Med* 60 (5): 379-86 (1993).

Gaucher, EJ and RJ Coffey. "A case study of quality improvement." in *Total Quality in Healthcare: From Theory to Practice (*San Francisco: Jossey-Bass, 1993), 397-440.

Willoughby, D, G Budreau, and D Livingston. "A framework for integrated quality improvement." *J Nurs Care Qual* 11 (3): 44–53.

Complying with Relevant JCAHO Standards

An emphasis on safety and systems analysis

With regard to medication safety, the healthcare industry is undergoing an important transformation. This book has focused on that transformation by exploring emergent strategies for improving the safety of medication use through systems analysis. But, for hospitals accredited by the Joint Commission on Accreditation of Healthcare Organizations (JCAHO), there's another, related side to medication use: compliance with relevant JCAHO standards. *(Editor's note: State laws, federal regulations, and the Health Care Financing Administration's "Conditions of Participation" also govern many of the issues and activities discussed here. Hospitals should consider all relevant requirements when developing medication-use policies and procedures.)* This chapter focuses on compliance with the JCAHO by: 1) reviewing the standards that affect medication use; 2) discussing "hot-button" compliance issues that, according to surveyors, pose problems for accredited organizations; and 3) outlining strategies for compliance.

But if this chapter shifts the book's focus, it does not necessarily redirect the book's gaze. The emphasis on safety and quality in the JCAHO standards often echoes the thinking behind the sentinel event policy and the systems-analysis approach to error prevention. The JCAHO standards manual acknowledges, for instance, that "medications are often essential to patient care,"[1] but it also stresses the risks of drug treatment and the importance of managing those risks by employing a standardized, systematic approach to medication use. It identifies medication use as a function that organizations must target for ongoing performance monitoring and improvement,[2] and it insists that these activities focus on underlying systems and processes, not on the actions and knowledge of individuals.[3] Complying with the JCAHO standards can be challenging and time consuming—even frustrating. But compliance and accreditation signal an organization's commitment to patient care and to progressive, systems-oriented methods for improving safety and quality that could have far-reaching effects on patient outcomes.

An overview of the relevant standards

Since the JCAHO reorganized its accreditation manual in 1994, standards that are relevant to medication use are sprinkled throughout. The largest concentration of relevant standards exists in the chapter on "Care of Patients" (TX), but organizations also will find standards that address medication use in the chapters on "Improving Organization Performance" (PI), "Management of Information" (IM), "Education" (PF), "Assessment of Patients" (PE), "Management of Human Resources" (HR), and "Medical Staff" (MS).

The JCAHO updates its manual quarterly, sometimes renumbering or slightly rewording standards. But it is less common for the underlying

---

[1] The Joint Commission on Accreditation of Healthcare Organizations, *Comprehensive Accreditation Manual for Hospitals (Oakbrook Terrace, IL: JCAHO, August 1997 update), TX-20. Subsequent references: CAMH, followed by relevant update and page-number information.*

[2] CAMH, *August 1998 update, PI-11.*

[3] CAMH, *August 1998 update, PI-1.*

goals of the standards to change significantly. To ensure that the information in this chapter remains as useful as possible, this discussion will focus on those underlying goals and will not identify standards by number. However, a list of relevant standard numbers appears in Appendix B, and updates to that list will be posted on the Opus Communications website *(www.opuscomm.com)* as the JCAHO releases them.

Care of Patients (TX)

The standards outlined in the chapter titled "Care of Patients" are designed to ensure that hospital staff work together to support the treatment goals and needs of patients. The JCAHO devotes a significant portion of this chapter to a discussion of medication use, emphasizing three main goals: 1) controlling access to medications; 2) maintaining the safety and effectiveness of drug treatment; and 3) monitoring outcomes of drug treatment. In emphasizing these goals, the JCAHO identifies five core processes within the medication-use function and designs standards to address each one. These core processes are: 1) selection, procurement, and storage; 2) prescribing and ordering; 3) preparation and dispensing; 4) administration; and 5) monitoring effects on the patient.[4]

Selection, procurement, and storage of medications

JCAHO expectations: The standards that address selection, procurement, and storage of medications call for the creation of a formulary—an inventory of drugs that an organization stocks and allows practitioners to prescribe. The JCAHO expects the development and maintenance of this formulary to be an ongoing, collaborative, and multi-disciplinary process that takes into account the needs of an

---

[4] CAMH, *August 1997 update, TX-20.*

organization's patient population as well as a drug's safety, effectiveness, and cost. However, the JCAHO recognizes that cases may arise in which a patient needs medication not on the formulary, and it expects organizations to establish effective policies and procedures for addressing these cases.

JCAHO surveyors also expect to see evidence that caregivers are familiar with safe and effective methods for storing medications, and that an organization takes steps to ensure that drugs are stored properly and securely. The standards do not assign one department responsibility for coordinating medication storage and control, but they imply that the pharmacy is probably best prepared to do so.

Compliance tips: To comply with the standards related to selection, procurement, and storage of medications, an organization should be prepared to show JCAHO surveyors a written copy of its formulary, along with documentation (e.g., meeting minutes) demonstrating that a multi-disciplinary task force—with representatives from the medical, pharmacy, nursing, and administrative staffs—reviews and considers changes to the formulary. In most hospitals, the pharmacy and therapeutics committee performs these reviews and submits formulary recommendations to the medical executive committee for consideration. An organization should have written policies that govern: 1) maintenance of the formulary; 2) procedures for ordering and procuring non-formulary medications; and 3) storage and control of medications. Clinical staff on the formulary-review task force and in patient-care areas should be familiar with these policies.

Hot-button issue: JCAHO surveyors say that they consistently see organizations struggle to control and store medications effectively—

especially on emergency crash carts, in operating rooms, and in night cabinets.

- **Crash carts:** Surveyors stress the importance of securing crash carts, and of inspecting them regularly to ensure they're adequately stocked and have remained secure. The JCAHO does not specify how often inspections should occur, allowing hospitals to schedule inspections at intervals that they consider appropriate. A safe rule of thumb—especially in critical care areas—is to have a nurse check cart contents and security once per shift. Organizations may want to have the pharmacy do a more extensive inspection each month. Organizations must be able demonstrate that they can identify every instance in which the lock or seal on a cart is broken. If they cannot do so they are technically unable to guarantee that a crash cart will be adequately stocked in an emergency. Hospitals often secure carts using break-away plastic locks on crash carts, which can be opened quickly in an emergency. Surveyors say that's fine, provided organizations number them or employ another reliable system for monitoring when locks are broken open and replaced. Organizations must also control access to replacement locks—even if locks are numbered. Storing locks where anyone can get at them is a violation because it makes it too easy to cover-up unauthorized use of a crash cart. One surveyor praised an organization that kept numbered break-away locks in its pharmacy. After a cart was opened and used, he said, it went immediately to the pharmacy, where staff restocked it, checked for expired or recalled medications, resealed the cart, logged the current lock number, and sent it back to the patient-care area. Whatever system an organization designs, it should have written policies that include a list of medications that can be stocked on carts, and that outline procedures for controlling cart contents (e.g., through inspections, use logs, etc.). It should also document cart inspections and restocking.

- **Operating rooms:** Surveyors say that operating rooms often pose control and storage problems because practitioners tend mistakenly to consider them "secure areas." Operating rooms are certainly more secure than some areas of a hospital, but staff who are not authorized to have access to medication (cleaning crews, maintenance workers, etc.) can enter operating rooms. Drugs sitting out in an operating room before or after a procedure are at risk of being stolen or misused. For instance, surveyors say it's not uncommon to find medication in unlabeled containers in operating rooms. If these containers are moved or switched (either maliciously or inadvertently), or if a practitioner becomes at all confused, the results can be tragic—as was the case for a seven-year-old boy in a Florida hospital. He died during routine ear surgery after being mistakenly injected with epinephrine—instead of lidocaine—from an unlabeled syringe. Hospitals that perform a lot of surgeries can often afford to staff satellite pharmacies in the OR, which means medication can be dispensed, as needed, during a procedure. Hospitals that cannot afford satellite pharmacies must have and enforce written policies about labeling and controlling medications in operating rooms. They should also seek to develop and document procedures for having drugs efficiently delivered to an OR during procedures (rather than having all medication delivered beforehand).

- **Night cabinets:** Surveyors noted that night cabinets are only an issue in organizations that do not staff a pharmacy 24 hours a day. The cabinets should contain a limited supply of drugs to be used when the pharmacy is closed. As with crash carts, JCAHO surveyors say

that organizations run into trouble if they don't have adequate policies and procedures for controlling access to the cabinets and for
regulating the supply of drugs stored in them. The pharmacy and
therapeutics committee or an equivalent body should determine
which medications are stored in night cabinets, based on likely need
and safety. The hospital should draft policies that are consistent with
relevant state law and that define who has the authority to remove
drugs from night cabinets. The hospital also should establish procedures to ensure that, when the pharmacy re-opens, a pharmacist
reviews all night-cabinet orders, restocks the cabinet, and can
determine who removed medication and how much was taken.
Technology exists that automatically tracks all relevant information
on night-cabinet use.

- **Other after-hours scenarios:** In addition to its night-cabinet requirements, the JCAHO expects organizations to develop policies and
  procedures that govern after-hours access to drugs that are not stored
  in a night cabinet. Often, access is limited to nurse supervisors, who
  can remove drugs in prepackaged, unit-dose containers from a
  secured area outside the pharmacy, or who can enter the pharmacy,
  itself, to retrieve medications. Hospitals also address after-hours dispensing by working with an off-site retail pharmacy that's open 24
  hours a day, which helps ensure pharmacist oversight of off-hours
  dispensing. However, hospitals that pursue such arrangements—or
  that use an off-site pharmacy for all drug dispensing, not just after-
  hours dispensing—should analyze state law carefully. In some states,
  licensing requirements are stricter for hospital pharmacists than for
  pharmacists working in retail outlets. If a hospital works with a retail
  pharmacy, JCAHO surveyors may ask if the retail pharmacists are
  licensed to work for a hospital. They also may ask the hospital to

describe its procedures for checking the credentials of those pharmacists.

Prescribing and ordering

JCAHO expectations: The JCAHO requires organizations to institute formal procedures for limiting risks associated with prescribing and ordering medication. The standards identify ten specific areas that organizations need to address (see Figure 5.1).

Compliance tips: Organizations need to have written policies that adequately address and govern each of the ten areas listed in Figure 5.1. Among other things, they need to be certain that these policies identify who can prescribe and order medications for patients (by law, this is limited to licensed physicians and, in some states, nurse practitioners and physician assistants), and that they outline guidelines and procedures regarding the maintenance, availability, and use of patient medication profiles (see Exhibit K, page 164).

Hot-button issue: Surveyors are likely to address any or all of the ten areas singled out in the JCAHO's standards manual, and each area presents its own challenges. However, surveyors say that control of sample drugs often proves especially problematic for organizations—particularly ambulatory clinics and other facilities that see outpatients.

Salespeople from pharmaceutical organizations supply samples, usually to familiarize physicians and patients with their products. Used correctly, samples can help doctors provide drug treatment for patients who don't have health insurance and can't afford to buy medicine; they also offer a means for determining whether a treatment regimen

Figure 5.1

Required prescription and ordering procedures

The JCAHO expects procedures supporting safe prescribing and ordering to address:

1. distribution and administration of controlled medications, including adequate documentation and recordkeeping required by law;

2   proper storage, distribution, and control of investigational medications and those in clinical trial;

3. situations in which all or some of a patient's medication orders must be permanently or temporarily canceled, and mechanisms for reinstating them;

4. "as needed" (PRN) prescriptions or orders and times of dose administration;

5. control of sample drugs;

6. distribution of medications to patients at discharge;

7. procurement, storage, control, and distribution of prepackaged medications obtained from outside sources;

8. procurement, storage, control, distribution, and administration of radioactive medications;

9. procurement, storage, control, distribution, administration, and monitoring of all blood derivatives; and

10. procurement, storage, control, distribution, administration, and monitoring of all radiographic contrast media.

Source: The Joint Commission on Accreditation of Healthcare Organizations, Comprehensive Accreditation Manual for Hospitals *(Oakbrook Terrace, IL: JCAHO, August 1997 update), TX-21.*

The patient medication profile

The patient medication profile (PMP) contains the specific information on a patient's condition, medical history, and medication treatment regimen that caregivers need to ensure the safety of that patient during drug treatment. Every patient who takes medication must have a PMP, and the PMP should be available to and easily accessed by pharmacy staff, nurses, and physicians. All staff involved in patient care should be able to add notations to the PMP, but only a pharmacist should have the authority and ability to change information in a PMP. Ideally, organizations make the PMP available by computer, which facilitates access and may allow more than one person to refer to a PMP simultaneously.

Following is a list of information that should generally appear in the PMP:

- the patient's name, birthdate, and gender;
- the patient's current height and weight;
- the patient's problems, symptoms, and/or diagnoses;
- all current medications a patient is taking—including investigational drugs;
- all known allergies and medication sensitivities;
- potential food-drug and/or drug-drug interactions;
- information, if relevant, on a patient's use of illegal drugs;
- information, if relevant, on a patient's misuse of prescription drugs;
- creatinine and BUN values for patients who are over 65 or candidates for kidney dysfunction; and
- body-surface area for chemotherapy patients.

As with all patient information, organizations should take steps to protect the confidentiality of medication profiles.

is effective before patients or insurers shoulder the cost of a full pre-scription. However, surveyors have found that organizations seem sometimes to forget that samples are subject to the same laws, regula-tions, and JCAHO standards that govern all medication: They must be stored securely; they can't be dispensed without a written order from a licensed, authorized practitioner; they can only be distributed by a physician or pharmacist; and organizations must track distribution and monitor effects.

Organizations that distribute samples should maintain sign-in and distribution logs for samples that, at the very least, include the informa-tion noted in Figure 5.2 (for sample log formats, see Figures 5.3 and 5.4, pages 167 and 168). As an article in the newsletter *Inside the Joint Commission* suggests, it's important to track batch numbers and patient names in case of a recall. The article suggests that including a physi-cian's signature and the name of the person who distributed the sample are crucial from a legal and accreditation standpoint. Having anyone other than a physician order medications, and anyone except a physi-cian or pharmacist distribute drugs, can be grounds for immediate revocation of accreditation. Likewise, nurses can lose their license for distributing samples. The article profiles a samples policy that includes the following requirements, and that reportedly satisfied the JCAHO:

1. No one, except the physician in charge of the clinic, can request non-formulary medications.
2. Practitioners dispensing samples must comply with all relevant state laws.
3. Staff must note distribution of all samples in a standardized log.
4. Physicians must document orders for and distribution of samples in a patient's medical record.[5]

---

[5] *"Require docs track sample meds to avoid Type Is"* Inside the Joint Commission, *May 4, 1998, 4-6.*

Figure 5.2

Recommended information for samples logs

Medication Sign-In Log	Medication Distribution Log
• the date the manufacturer provided the samples	• the names of patients receiving the samples
• the drug name	• the dosage and number of doses given to each patient
• the manufacturer's lot number	
• the number of sample doses received	• the manufacturer's lot or batch number
• the expiration date for the lot	• the signature of the physician that prescribed or ordered the samples
• name and signature of the person who accepted the samples	• the name and position of the person who distributed the samples

Preparation and dispensing

JCAHO expectations: These standards apply most directly to pharmacy practices. JCAHO expects organizations to comply with all laws, regulations, and practice standards governing the preparation and dispensing of medications and the licensing of individuals who prepare

Figure 5.3

Samples sign-in log

Date Rec'd	Drug Name (Brand & Generic)	Manufacturer's Lot Number	Amount Rec'd	Exp. Date	Person Making Log Entry (Name & Signature)

Source: Opus Communications, "Free sample drugs come with a price," Briefings on JCAHO/AAAHC: *Ambulatory Care, May 1998, 10.*

Figure 5.4

Log of sample medications dispensed

Sample medications dispensed

Drug Name (Brand & Generic):

Date Disp'd	Patient Name	Medical Record #	Lot Number	Exp. Date	# of Doses	Dispensed by* (Name & Signature)	Signature of Ordering LIP*

*Only physicians and pharmacists can dispense medication to patients. No medication can be dispensed without a written order signed by the patient's physician or another authorized LIP (licensed independent practitioner).

and dispense drugs. Surveyors will also want to see evidence that organizations:

- employ standardized dosing, distribution, and labeling procedures to help prevent medication errors;
- dispense medication in the most ready-to-administer form
  possible;
- have procedures for preventing patients from receiving expired
  medications; and
- have pharmacists review all prescriptions and medication
  orders (except in specific clinical and emergency situations).[6]

The JCAHO insists that diagnoses, known allergies, and other patient information be available to support reviews of prescriptions. It also wants this information available so people involved in preparing and dispensing medication can 1) facilitate continuity of care; 2) create an accurate medication history; 3) supplement monitoring of [adverse drug events]; and 4) provide safe administration of medications.[7]

Finally, the JCAHO expects organizations to have effective procedures in place for tracking dispensed medications—including samples (see page 162)—in case of a discontinuation or recall.

Compliance tips: To comply with standards governing the preparation and dispensing of drugs, the JCAHO recommends that hospitals dispense drugs in the most ready-to-administer form possible. The *CAMH* cites use of unit-dose distribution as one possible approach to compliance. Many organizations now use unit-dose distribution, but they

---

[6] CAMH, *August 1997 update, TX-22.*

[7] *Ibid.*

should also have written policies and procedures to support and facilitate that system and to:

- define who has the authority to prepare and dispense medication;
- outline standardized procedures for labeling medication in all preparation areas, including satellite pharmacies;
- mandate that a pharmacist review and initial orders and prescriptions, and to define the scope of these reviews;
- describe the information that must be noted in a patient's chart and medication profile to facilitate pharmacist reviews; and
- explain procedures for inspecting drug stocks to ensure patients do not receive expired, recalled, or discontinued medications.

Hospitals should keep copies of relevant policies, laws, and regulations in the pharmacy and in other areas where medication is prepared and dispensed. They should address this information and accepted standards of practice during training and inservice sessions for staff who are authorized to prepare and dispense medications, and document the information covered and attendance at these sessions.

Organizations should periodically inspect a sampling of medication orders and patient charts to confirm that staff are complying with relevant policies, and to ensure that orders are supported by appropriate chart documentation. Those inspections should be documented in writing, and inspection reports should be presented as evidence of compliance during a JCAHO survey.

Hot-button issue: Monitoring for expired, recalled, and discontinued medications is an area that, according to JCAHO surveyors, consistently causes problems for organizations. They say pharmacy staff should inspect drug stocks monthly, replace drugs as needed, and carefully document their work and findings.

- **Recalls and discontinuations:** As with drug samples, staff should log the manufacturer lot numbers on all medications stored in pharmacy stocks, night cabinets, medication carts, and elsewhere on units (e.g., floor stocks). For each dose that's dispensed to a patient, staff should log both the lot number and the name of the patient who receives the medication. These logs will allow an organization quickly to track medication in the event of a recall or discontinuation. They will also serve as evidence of compliance during a JCAHO survey.

- **Expired medications:** Surveyors suggest that organizations use stickers to make inspections for expired medications easier and more effective. These stickers, they say, go on the outside of a medication cupboard or drawer and indicate when the next drug in that cupboard or drawer will expire, reducing the likelihood that expiration dates get overlooked and patients receive expired medication.

Administration

JCAHO expectations: The standards that apply to medication administration affect the nursing and medical staffs most directly. They are designed to ensure that properly trained and licensed individuals administer medications to patients, that those people verify orders and patient identification before administering drugs, and that they take other steps to augment the safety and effectiveness of drug treatment. In addition to general medication use, these standards address procedures and policies for dealing with investigational medications and medications that patients bring with them to a hospital.

Compliance tips: These standards address what are sometimes called the "five rights" of medication use: right patient, right drug, right dose, right time, and right route of administration. Organizations should have written policies mandating verification of this information, and requiring staff to document verification. They should also design and document training and inservice sessions to support these policies. Hospitals might want to consider employing bar coding and other technologies to support and improve the accuracy of verification and identification activities (see page 43 for more on bar coding).

Beyond verification activities, these standards require hospitals to design "alternative medication administration systems" for medications that patients bring with them to a hospital and/or that they will be administering to themselves. If, upon admission to a hospital, patients are on medication, the organization should have procedures in place for factoring that existing regimen into all decisions regarding additional medication use. A physician must assess all medications that patients bring with them to the facility—to determine whether use of the drugs is medically appropriate. If patients bring controlled substances or prescription medications to the hospital, the hospital must confirm that written orders authorize use of the drugs; organizations should have a written policy requiring this confirmation. If patients will be self-administering medications, the organizations should have written policies that outline procedures for ensuring that patients understand how to administer their medications and for supporting safe, effective self-administration.

Hot-button issue: Surveyors say that they're careful to ensure that organizations prevent unlicensed or unauthorized individuals from administering medication. One surveyor said that's particularly true for drugs used in "conscious sedation."

That surveyor also noted that the emergence of healthcare networks is forcing organizations to wrestle with new issues. For instance, in California, where this surveyor is based, physician's assistants can administer medication in independent clinics and physician's offices, but not in hospitals or any facility that's part of a hospital-based network. Following a merger, therefore, hospital-based networks in California must hold clinics to the medication-administration standards that govern hospitals. State laws on this and related issues vary, said the surveyor, so organizations involved in mergers and acquisitions must be familiar with the nuances of relevant laws and regulations and adjust policies and procedures, as needed.

Monitoring the effects of medication on patients

JCAHO expectations: The current standard that requires organizations continually to assess the effects of medication is designed to ensure that monitoring activities are inter-disciplinary and interactive. They insist that physicians, pharmacists, and nurses work together to monitor effects, that they rely on information in medical records and patient medication profiles, and that they seek input from patients and their families.

Compliance tips: All monitoring activities must be documented in patient medical records, and organizations should have written policies and procedures that address JCAHO requirements and that govern drug-effects monitoring. These documents should mandate collaboration between physicians, nurses, and pharmacists, should create channels that facilitate and guide this collaboration, and should require caregivers to seek patient input. Among other things, hospital policies and procedures should provide the means for:

- pharmacists to question medication orders that seem inconsistent with aspects of patient diagnoses and/or medication profiles;

- nurses to question abnormal doses or pharmacy deliveries that seem inconsistent with medication orders; and

- nurses, physicians, or pharmacists to report the effects of drug treatment, including unexpected outcomes and adverse drug events.

Hot-button issue: Failure to document monitoring activities can undermine otherwise effective monitoring programs and can place an organization's accreditation status in jeopardy. Simply presenting effective policy and procedure documents is not enough; JCAHO surveyors expect to see evidence that staff comply with those policies and that hospital leaders enforce them. Organizations should design training and inservice sessions to help improve the effectiveness of caregiver documentation, and they should require staff in the health information management department to return charts to caregivers when documentation is inadequate.

Improving Organization Performance (PI)

The PI standards are meant to ensure that an "organization designs processes well and systematically monitors, analyzes, and improves its performance to improve patient outcomes."[8] These standards require

---

[8] CAMH, *August 1998 update, PI-1.*

organizations to collect performance data on critical hospital functions and launch improvement initiatives based on that data. Because medication-use processes are often central to patient care and can be closely associated with patient outcomes, many PI standards have some link to medication use. However, this discussion will focus on standards that single out medication use or sentinel events (medication-related incidents being a leading cause of sentinel events—see page 64) as a target for data-driven performance improvement.

Processes that hospitals must monitor

JCAHO expectations: The JCAHO counts medication use among the six processes that organizations are required to monitor, because these processes "are known to be high-risk, high-volume, or problem-prone

---

Figure 5.5

High-risk, high-volume, problem-prone processes

Organizations select performance measures for processes that are known to jeopardize the safety of the individuals served or [are] associated with sentinel events in similar health care organizations. At a minimum, the organization identifies performance measures related to the following processes, as appropriate to the care and services provided:

1. Medication use;
2. Operative and other procedures that place patients at risk;
3. Use of blood and blood components;
4. Restraint use;
5. Seclusion when it is part of the care or services provided; and
6. Care or services provided to high-risk populations

Source: The Joint Commission on Accreditation of Healthcare Organizations, Comprehensive Accreditation Manual for Hospitals *(Oakbrook Terrace, IL: JCAHO, August 1998 update), PI-11 (PI.3.1.1).*

---

areas related to the care and services provided"[9] (see Figure 5.5). The standards allow organizations to choose their own "performance measures," to decide how frequently they will collect data, and to decide how detailed that data will be. However, the standards clearly indicate that these activities need to be rigorous enough to "identify opportunities for improvement, identify changes that will lead to improvement, and sustain improvement."[10]

Compliance tips: Organizations should assess their patient populations and treatment trends to identify which high-risk, high-volume, and problem-prone areas of medication use they are most justified in monitoring. Then they should develop written policies that clearly define organizational performance measures, collection tools and techniques, and monitoring requirements. They should have an inter-disciplinary task force (e.g., the pharmacy and therapeutics committee) review medication-use data and identify improvement opportunities. And they should document the results of improvement initiatives.

Sentinel-event monitoring

JCAHO expectations: The JCAHO PI standards that address sentinel events cite "significant medication errors" and "significant adverse drug reactions" among the incidents that organizations must investigate (see Figure 5.6).[11] In addition to incidents that meet the JCAHO's definition of "sentinel event," ("an unexpected occurrence or variation involving death or serious physical or psychological injury, or the risk thereof"[12]),

---

[9] CAMH, *August 1998 update, PI-11.*

[10] CAMH, *August 1998 update, PI-9.*

[11] CAMH, *August 1998 update, PI-17.*

[12] *Joint Commission on Accreditation of Healthcare Organizations,* Sentinel Events: Evaluating Cause and Planning Improvement *(Oakbrook Terrace, IL: JCAHO, 1998), 7.*

Figure 5.6

Events requiring root-cause analysis

- Confirmed transfusion reactions
- Significant adverse drug reactions
- Significant medication errors
- Major discrepancies, or patterns of discrepancies, between preoperative and postoperative diagnoses; and
- Significant adverse events associated with anesthesia use

Source: Joint Commission on Accreditation of Healthcare Organizations.

these standards require organizations to analyze instances and patterns of performance that: 1) don't live up to internal expectations; 2) lag behind performance at other healthcare organizations; and 3) are out of sync with recognized standards of care. The JCAHO standards require organizations to use the results of their analysis to improve performance and lessen the risk of future sentinel events (see Chapters 3 and 4 for more on investigating sentinel events and designing systems improvements). These standards seem designed to support many of the goals of the JCAHO's sentinel event policy and to compel healthcare organizations to apply the systems-analysis approach to error prevention to a wider range of incidents than sentinel events, as the JCAHO defines them.

Compliance tips: Organizations must have written policies that define what they consider to be events meriting root-cause analysis (see Chapter 3 for more on root-cause analysis), or that explain their process for deciding when to investigate incidents or patterns of performance variation. They should also have clearly defined procedures for collecting performance data (for all JCAHO-mandated processes and functions and others that they deem relevant), and for comparing their performance with internal expectations, industry benchmarks, and accepted standards. They should hold and document training sessions to educate staff about the tools and techniques of root-cause analysis and performance/quality improvement, documenting these sessions and the results of actual improvement initiatives.

The leadership component

To be truly successful, performance-improvement initiatives and root-cause analyses must have the backing and authority of organizational leadership. The JCAHO recognizes this—which is why its PI standards have a strong leadership component, and why it has added a sentinel event standard to the "Leadership" chapter in the CAMH (the LD standards).

The PI standards require organizational leaders to "establish a planned, systematic, organization-wide approach to process design and to performance measurement, analysis, and improvement."[13] The leadership standard requires hospital leaders to "ensure that the processes for identifying and managing sentinel events are defined and implemented."[14] It also requires leaders to establish "process for the identification, reporting, analysis, and prevention of sentinel events, and for ensuring the consistent and effective implementation of a mechanism to accomplish these activities."[15]

---

[13] CAMH, *August 1998 update, PI-5.*

[14] *Opus Communications, "Sentinel event standard may appear in Leadership chapter next year,"* Briefings on JCAHO, *August 1998, 2. And* CAMH, *November 1998 update, LD-36a.*

[15] CAMH, *November 1998 update, LD-36a.*

Management of Information (IM)

Because management of information plays a crucial role in providing quality care and improving organizational performance, many of the JCAHO's IM standards have a link to medication use. This discussion will focus on instances in which that link is stated explicitly or strongly implied.

Documenting medication use

JCAHO expectations: The JCAHO requires organizations to document, among other things, the following information on medication use in patient medical records:

- every medication order or prescription;
- every dose of medication administered;
- every adverse drug reaction; and
- all medications dispensed to ambulatory patients or to inpatients on discharge.

JCAHO's IM standards also require postoperative documentation to note all medications administered during a procedure, including intravenous fluids. For outpatients, they require organizations to maintain a "summary list" in each patient's medical record that notes, among other things, significant drug allergies and medications; that list is required to appear in the patients' medical record no later than their third visit to a facility.[16]

Compliance tips: Organizations should have written policies that define their requirements regarding chart documentation, order authentication, progress notes, and summary lists. These policies should address

---

[16] CAMH, *August 1997 update, IM-20–IM-23.*

each of the JCAHO's explicit requirements and expectations. Organizations should assess medication-use documentation as part of the ongoing-record–review process, and they should hold training sessions to ensure that HIM analysts and coders review chart documentation effectively. They should also develop and enforce policies and procedures to ensure that the HIM and medical staffs work together to clarify insufficient chart documentation.

Collecting and analyzing aggregate data on medication use

JCAHO expectations: The JCAHO standards acknowledge that the documentation in patient medical records (and information in other sources and databases) can play an important role in assessing the overall quality of care at an organization and in designing performance-improvement initiatives. To facilitate these processes, the IM standards require organizations to collect and analyze aggregate data on a range of functions, processes, outcomes, and other core activities, and they specifically mention two aspects of medication use: 1) transactions in the pharmacy, "as required by law and to control and account for all drugs"; and 2) key information on the receipt, use, and disposal of radionuclides and radiopharmaceuticals.[17]

The IM standards also require aggregation and analysis of data and information on outcomes- and process-related performance measures. The IM chapter does not single out medication use as a required focus of these collection and analysis activities, but the PI chapter (see page 174) does. Considered in the context of the JCAHO's PI standards, therefore, the link between medication use and the requirements for aggregation of data are strong; personnel responsible for ensuring compliance with these requirements should be thoroughly familiar with the medication-use aspects of the PI standards.

---

[17] CAMH, *August and November 1997 updates, IM-34–IM-35.*

Compliance tips: Organizations should have written policies that describe requirements and procedures for aggregating and analyzing patient- and treatment-related information. These policies should address the aspects of medication use covered explicitly in the IM standards, and they should take into account relevant links to medication-use requirements in other areas of the *CAMH*—most notably the PI chapter. Hospitals should establish vehicles for aggregating and analyzing relevant data (e.g., a chart-review task force, monitoring software, etc.), and they should document all monitoring and improvement activities.

Education (PF)

The PF standards acknowledge the crucial role that patients and patients' families play in treatment. In general, these standards seek to ensure that organizations involve patients and their families in treatment-related decisions and activities, and that organizations provide patients and their families with the information and training they need to be effective participants and decision-makers.

Education and medication use

JCAHO expectations: The JCAHO's standards require that organizations educate patients and families about safe, effective, and legal medication use. In providing this education, organizations are expected to take into account important variables like:

- the patient's and family's beliefs and values;
- literacy, educational level, and language;
- emotional barriers and motivations;
- physical and cognitive limitations; and
- the financial implications of care choices.[18]

---

[18] CAMH, *August 1997 update*, PF-5–PF-7.

Regardless of whether a patient is self-administering medications, education should ensure that patients and key family members understand basic information that is crucial to effective medication use, including: the name(s) of the drug(s) they are taking, the dosage(s), the dosing schedule, whether the medication(s) should be taken on a full or empty stomach, and whether the drug(s) should not be taken with certain foods or certain other drugs. It should also cover topics that will help patients provide information on the effectiveness of drug treatment, including: common side effects, expected benefits, circumstances or effects that warrant a patient calling a doctor or pharmacist, and possible food-drug or drug-drug interactions.

Compliance tips: An organization's written medication-use policies should address patient and family education and clearly define the educational responsibilities of caregivers. In addition, organizations should stress to clinical staff the importance of documenting educational activities in a patient's chart. To ensure that documentation meets JCAHO expectations, hospitals should make evaluation of relevant documentation a regular component of ongoing record review.

Hot-button issue: Surveyors say that hospitals consistently have trouble satisfying JCAHO requirements regarding education about possible food-drug interactions. If they haven't done so already, organizations might consider creating programs specifically to address this issue. Among other things, the program could identify the most common and dangerous food-drug interactions and address practical ways that patients can modify their diets to avoid interactions while still maintaining proper nutrition. Involving all relevant disciplines—physicians, nurses, pharmacists, and dietitians—is the most effective approach to education. Members of the pharmacy and therapeutics committee and nutrition staff should help draft and/or review all educational materials developed for the program.

Assessment of Patients (PE)

JCAHO expectations: The PE standards require an organization to assess, among other things, the physical status of patients that it admits. This assessment can take place within a time frame that the organization determines after considering a range of factors, including: "the types of patients treated by the hospital, the complexity and duration of their care, and the dynamics of conditions surrounding their care."[19] However, a patient's medical history, physical examination, nursing assessment, and any screening assessments must be completed within 24 hours of admission. The history and physical is particularly relevant to medication use because it includes an overview of a patient's medication history, including current medications and known allergies.

Once treatment begins, organizations are required to reassess a patient at regular intervals and whenever a change in condition warrants. These reassessments should:

- determine the patient's response to care, including his or her response to drug treatment; and
- identify, prioritize, and/or adjust aspects of treatment, including medication use, based on the patient's specific needs.

The JCAHO expects assessments and reassessments to be collaborative and multi-disciplinary, allowing caregivers to integrate information and views to improve the overall quality of care.

---

[19] CAMH, *August 1997 update, PE-8–PE-9.*

Compliance tips: Organizations need to have clear policies addressing each of the JCAHO's requirements regarding patient assessments. They should review chart documentation to ensure that assessment activities comply with those policies and the JCAHO's standards.

Management of Human Resources (HR)

The *CAMH* chapter titled "Management of Human Resources" addresses issues related to staff size, competency, training, and continuing education. Medication use is not mentioned specifically, but because these standards address the qualifications and ability of staff to perform patient-care activities—including, presumably, those associated with medication use—they are relevant to this book.

Medication-use competency and staff education

JCAHO expectations: The standards require hospital leaders to define qualifications and performance expectations for the staff, and to ensure that an organization employs an appropriate number of qualified people. These standards also require organizations to encourage staff self-development and to support monitoring, orientation, and training programs that assess staff competency levels, target competency needs, and/or improve the competency of the overall staff and of individual staff members.[20]

Compliance tips: In the context of medication use, organizations should have policies that define who on the staff can prescribe, order, dispense, and/or administer medications; these policies must be consistent with all relevant laws, regulations, and standards. Organizations should document staff compliance with, and organizational enforcement of,

---

[20] CAMH, *May and November updates, HR-5–HR-11, HR-13–HR-19.*

these policies. They should also be prepared to discuss orientation, training, and inservice procedures, and to show evidence of a commitment to staff orientation, training, assessment, and other activities designed to measure and improve staff competency.

Medical Staff (MS)

As with the HR standards, the links between medication use and the standards in the *CAMH* chapter titled "Medical Staff" are clear, but largely indirect. This discussion will focus on the MS standards that are most relevant to medication use.

Medication use, privileges, and patient care

JCAHO expectations: Perhaps the most notable link between the MS standards and medication use are the standards governing credentialing, privileging, and patient-care activities. The following requirements apply:

- Hospitals must ensure that licensed independent practitioners (LIP) manage all aspects of patient care (including drug treatment). However, LIP can only provide treatment and perform procedures that lie within the scope of the clinical privileges the hospital grants them. *(Editor's note: The issue of privileges is particularly relevant to medication use in states that allow some nonphysician LIP—e.g., nurse practitioners or physician assistants—to prescribe drugs. Hospitals usually do not let these practitioners prescribe without specific privileges. It's less common for hospitals to require physicians to secure prescribing privileges—though some hospitals do, especially for high-risk medications. As used here, LIP denotes physicians and some nonphysicians, but the scenarios discussed tend most often to affect nonphysician practitioners.)*

• Hospitals also must have a defined credentialing process in place for: 1) appointing and reappointing properly LIP to the medical staff; and 2) granting, reviewing, and revising clinical privileges (including, where relevant, prescribing privileges). These privileges must be specific to that individual and that hospital, and they must clearly define the limitations on that individual's authority to treat or direct treatment.

• Hospitals must have mechanisms in place to ensure that an LIP's patient-care activities do not exceed the scope of his or her privileges.

• The standards allow organizations to develop their own mechanisms for reviewing and granting privileges, and for monitoring compliance with privileges, provided these mechanisms are in accordance with state law. However, the JCAHO expects hospitals to demonstrate that privileging decisions are based on an assessment of a practitioner's current competence, taking into account: 1) the individual's relevant documented experience; 2) applicable results and outcomes from his or her treatment history; and 3) data and conclusions from pertinent performance-improvement initiatives. A practitioner's board-certification status should also factor into privileging decisions.

Compliance tips: An organization's medical staff policies, bylaws, and related documents should define its process for validating LIP qualifications before securing or renewing privileges. Minimum qualifications generally include license and registration, confirmation of training that is consistent with a clinical privileges request (e.g., residencies and clinical practice experience with a track record of successful treatment), and/or board certification. Participation in continuing-education (CE) programs demonstrates a practitioner's commitment to maintaining and/or improving competency, so organizations should demonstrate that CE factors into decisions regarding reappointment to the medical staff and renewal or revision of privileges.

An organization's policies and bylaws should outline point-of-service procedures that are used to check LIP privileges before treatment is provided. Furthermore, documentation in patient charts and other databases should demonstrate that staff employ these checks. For instance, before pharmacists approve a medication order (particularly one written by a nonphysician LIP), organizations might require them to document that they have confirmed that a practitioner's privileges permit treatment of the diagnosed condition.

The importance of continuing education

JCAHO expectations: Research has suggested that many medication errors and adverse drug reactions could be prevented if practitioners had more information on the drugs involved (see Chapters 1 and 2). There are too many drugs on the market, and too many drug-treatment variables, for organizations to expect practitioners to know and remember everything about the drugs they prescribe. Nonetheless, it's crucial for members of the medical staff to be as knowledgeable as possible about medications, and to seek to expand their knowledge base. That's why the JCAHO's MS standards on continuing medical education (CME) are relevant to medication use. The standards require all individuals with clinical privileges to participate in CME activities, and they require organizations to document this participation. They also require hospitals to sponsor CME activities that relate 1) to the type and nature of care provided in a facility; and 2) to performance-improvement findings that reveal training/CME needs.

Compliance tips: CME has been an integrated component of health-care for a long time, and most organizations already offer the medical staff access to educational forums. It's important, however, to keep a record of attendance at CME functions as documentation of participation. It's also important to ensure that some of the CME programs that an organization sponsors address needs identified by performance-improvement initiatives. Case presentations, summaries of articles from medical journals, and lectures by visiting professors are all tried and true approaches to CME.

The medical staff's role in performance improvement

JCAHO expectations: The MS standards require the medical staff to lead improvement initiatives that address clinical processes that are the primary responsibility of physicians. They single out assessment and improvement of medication use as specific areas, among others, that require medical-staff leadership.[21] The standards also require the medical staff to participate in (though not necessarily to lead) multi-disciplinary initiatives seeking to improve other patient-care processes.

Compliance tips: These aspects of the MS standards are closely associated with the chapter on "Improving Organization Performance" (the PI standards), with the new standards on sentinel events in the PI and "Leadership" chapters, and with the JCAHO's controversial sentinel event policy. Individuals responsible for ensuring compliance with the

---

[21] CAMH, *August 1998 update, MS-48–MS-49.*

MS standards should also be familiar with the JCAHO's broader expectations regarding performance improvement and sentinel events.

To ensure compliance with these components of the MS standards, organizational policies should require all PI initiatives to be multi-disciplinary—involving, whenever possible, physicians, pharmacists, and nurses. And they must clearly define the kinds of initiatives that require medical-staff leadership—like, for instance, those addressing adverse drug reactions, medication-related sentinel events, and other medication-use issues or topics. Organizations should be sure to document their performance-improvement activities and the medical staff's involvement in those initiatives.

Accepting the patient-safety challenge

Drug treatment can be complex and risky, but it's also an indispensable component of patient care. Recognizing both its dangers and its potential benefits, the JCAHO has molded and regularly reviews accreditation standards that are designed to help organizations manage the medication-use process and prevent adverse events and outcomes. The standards stress the importance of having well-trained, licensed individuals involved in each stage of the process—from ordering and dispensing to administering and effects monitoring. But they also acknowledge that well-trained, well-intentioned individuals need support, emphasizing: 1) the importance of caregiver collaboration during each stage of medication use; 2) the value of systemic checks and balances to support that collaboration; and 3) the significance of performance monitoring and continuous improvement.

In this context, the link between the JCAHO standards and the systems-analysis approach to error prevention seems clear. Both operate under the assumption that, while individuals carry some responsibility for error prevention, it's bad systems—not bad people—that most often cause problems during drug treatment. Both also recognize that, to reduce the tragic impact of medication errors and adverse drug events, healthcare organizations must abandon blame-oriented response strategies and focus prevention efforts at the systemic level. In the past few years, healthcare innovators have taken important strides in this direction; the challenge now lies in sustaining their momentum and in building on the foundation that they have laid.

SUGGESTED READING

Books

Barnard, Cynthia and Jodi L. Eisenberg. *Performance Improvement: Winning Strategies for Quality and JCAHO Compliance* (Marblehead, MA: Opus Communications, 1998).

Chamberlain, Kathryn, Jay Coburn, and Jodi L. Eisenberg. *The JCAHO Survey Coordinator's Handbook* (Marblehead, MA: Opus Communications, 1997).

Chamberlain, Kathryn and Candace Hamner. *The JCAHO Mock Survey Made Simple* (Marblehead, MA: Opus Communications, 1998).

Cofer, Jennifer I., Hugh Greeley, and Jay Coburn. *Information Management: The Compliance Guide to the JCAHO Standards* (Marblehead, MA: Opus Communications, 1998).

Hamner, Candace. *Ready, Set, JCAHO! Questions, Games, and Other Strategies to Prepare Your Staff for Survey* (Marblehead, MA: Opus Communications, 1998).

Iacono, Joan and Ann Campbell. *Patient and Family Education: The Compliance Guide to the JCAHO Standards* (Marblehead, MA: Opus Communications, 1997).

Thompson, Richard E. *The Compliance Guide to the Medical Staff Standards: Winning Strategies for your JCAHO Survey* (Marblehead, MA: Opus Communications, 1998).

Articles

Schaff, RL, et al. "Development of the Joint Commission's Indicators for Monitoring the Medication Use System." *Hosp Pharm* 26: 326-30 (1991).

Other Resources

Reporting programs for adverse drug events:

JCAHO Sentinel Event Hotline

(630) 792-3700

www.jcaho.org

Medwatch: The FDA Medical Products Reporting Program

(800) FDA-1088 (332-1088)

www.fda.gov/medwatch

Practitioners' Reporting Network (US Pharmacopeia):

- Medication Errors Reporting Program
  (800) 23-ERROR (233-7767)
  www.usp.org/practrep/mer.htm

- Drug Product Problem Reporting Program
  (800) 4-USP-PRN (487-7776)
  www.usp.org/practrep/dppr.htm

- Drug Product Problem Reporting Program for
  Radiopharmaceuticals
  (800) 4-USP-PRN (487-7776)
  www.usp.org/practrep/radio.htm

Organizations that address patient and medication safety

American Pharmaceutical Association

2215 Constitution Avenue, NW

Washington, DC 20037-2985

(202) 628-4410

www.aphanet.org

American Society of Health-System Pharmacists

7272 Wisconsin Avenue

Bethesda, MD 20814

(301) 657-3000

www.ashp.org

The Anesthesia Patient Safety Foundation

c/o Mercy Hospital

1400 Locust Street

Pittsburgh, PA 15219-5166

(412) 281-9484

gasnet.med.yale.edu/societies/apsf

Institute for Healthcare Improvement

135 Francis Street

Boston, MA 02215

(617) 754-4800

www.ihi.org

The Institute for Safe Medication Practices

300 West Street Road

Warminster, PA 18974-3236

(215) 956-9181

www.ismp.org

Joint Commission on Accreditation of Healthcare Organizations

One Renaissance Boulevard

Oakbrook Terrace, IL 60181

(630) 792-5000

www.jcaho.org

National Association for Healthcare Quality

4700 W. Lake Avenue

Glenview, IL 60025

(800) 966-9392

www.nahq.org

The National Patient Safety Foundation at the AMA

515 North State Street, 8th Floor

Chicago, IL 60610

(312) 464-4848

www.ama-assn.org/med-sci/npsf

US Pharmacopeia

12601 Twinbrook Parkway

Rockville, MD 20852

(800) 822-8772

www.usp.org

JCAHO Standards on Medication Use

Relevant standard numbers

The discussion in Chapter 5 is based on analysis of the standards listed in the table that follows. These standard numbers come from the JCAHO's *Comprehensive Accreditation Manual for Hospitals (CAMH)*; quarterly updates through the third quarter of 1998 are covered. If, in future quarterly updates, the JCAHO renumbers these standards or makes other relevant revisions to its manual, Opus Communications will post updates on its Internet site: *www.opuscomm.com*.

Care of patients (TX)

TX.3	TX.3.4	TX.3.5.3	TX.3.6
TX.3.1	TX.3.5	TX.3.5.4	TX.3.7
TX.3.2	TX.3.5.1	TX.3.5.5	TX.3.8
TX.3.3	TX.3.5.2	TX.3.5.6	TX.3.9

Improving organization performance (PI)

PI.1	PI.3.1.1	PI.4.4
PI.3.1	PI.4.3	

Leadership (LD)

LD.4.3.4

Management of information (IM)

IM.7	IM.7.3.3	IM.7.4.1
IM.7.2	IM.7.4	IM.8

Education (PF)

PF.1.3	PF.1.5

Assessment of patients (PE)

PE.1	PE.1.6.1	PE.2.1	PE.2.3	PE.3
PE.1.6	PE.2	PE.2.2	PE.2.4	PE.3.1

Management of human resources (HR)

HR.1	HR.3	HR.4	HR.4.3
HR.2	HR.3.1	HR.4.2	HR.5

Medical staff (MS)

MS.5.14	MS.5.15.1.2	MS.7.1	MS.7.2.1
MS.5.14.1	MS.5.15.1.3	MS.7.1.1	MS.8
MS.5.14.2	MS.5.15.2	MS.7.1.1.1	MS.8.1
MS.5.15	MS.5.15.3	MS.7.1.1.2	MS.8.1.2
MS.5.15.1	MS.7	MS.7.2	MS.8.2
MS.5.15.1.1			

Related Products from Opus Communications

Newsletters

Briefings on Adverse and Sentinel Events

Briefings on Assisted Living

Briefings on Behavioral Health Accreditation

Briefings on Credentialing

Briefings on Hospital Safety

Briefings on Laboratory Safety and Accreditation

Briefings on Long-Term Care Regulations

Briefings on JCAHO

Briefings on JCAHO: Home Health and Hospice

Briefings on JCAHO/AAAHC: Ambulatory Care

Credentialing Across the Continuum

Executive Briefings on Health Care Regulations

Health Governance Report

Long-Term Care Survey Monitor

Medical Staff Briefing

Physician Practice Compliance Report

Books

The Compliance Guide to the Medical Staff Standards, second edition

The Credentialing Desk Reference, second edition

Credentialing Without Complexity

Effective Communication for the Medical Staff

The Greeley Guide to Medical Staff Credentialing

The Greeley Guide to Managed Care Credentialing

A Guide to Centralized Credentialing

Information Management: The Compliance Guide to the JCAHO Standards, second edition

The JCAHO Home Health Mock Survey Made Simple, 1999 edition

The JCAHO Mock Survey Made Simple, 1999 edition

The JCAHO Survey Coordinator's Handbook, second edition

Leadership: The Compliance Guide to the JCAHO Standards

The Medical Staff Leaders' Practical Guide, third edition

Patient and Family Education: The Compliance Guide to the JCAHO Standards

Performance Improvement: Winning Strategies for Quality and JCAHO Compliance

Quality Improvement Techniques for Hospital Safety

Quality Improvement Techniques for Long-Term Care

Quality Improvement Techniques for Respiratory Care

Ready, Set, JCAHO! Questions, Games, and Other Strategies to Prepare Your Staff for Survey

Restraint and Seclusion: Improving Practice and Conquering the JCAHO Standards

Streamlining Quality Monitoring

The Top Twenty Medical Staff Policies and Procedures